Nursing in Partnership with Patients and Carers

Transforming Nursing Practice series

Transforming Nursing Practice is the first series of books designed to help students meet the requirements of the NMC Standards and Essential Skills Clusters for degree programmes. Each book addresses a core topic, and together they cover the generic knowledge required for all fields of practice. Accessible and challenging, *Transforming Nursing Practice* helps nursing students prepare for the demands of future healthcare delivery.

Core knowledge titles:

Series editor: Dr Shirley Bach, Head of the School of Nursing and Midwifery at the University of Brighton

Communication and Interpersonal Skills in Nursing (2nd. ed)	ISBN 978 0 85725 449 8
Contexts of Contemporary Nursing (2nd. ed.)	ISBN 978 1 84445 374 0
Health Promotion and Public Health for Nursing Students	ISBN 978 0 85725 437 5
Introduction to Medicines Management in Nursing	ISBN 978 1 84445 845 5
Law and Professional Issues in Nursing (2nd. ed.)	ISBN 978 1 84445 372 6
Leadership, Management and Team Working in Nursing	ISBN 978 0 85725 453 5
Learning Skills for Nursing Students	ISBN 978 1 84445 376 4
Medicines Management in Adult Nursing	ISBN 978 1 84445 842 4
Medicines Management in Children's Nursing	ISBN 978 1 84445 470 9
Medicines Management in Mental Health Nursing	ISBN 978 0 85725 049 0
Nursing Adults with Long Term Conditions	ISBN 978 0 85725 441 2
Nursing and Collaborative Practice (2nd. ed)	ISBN 978 1 84445 373 3
Nursing and Mental Health Care	ISBN 978 1 84445 467 9
Passing Calculations Tests for Nursing Students	ISBN 978 1 84445 471 6
Patient and Carer Participation in Nursing	ISBN 978 0 85725 307 1
Successful Practice Learning for Nursing Students (2nd. ed)	ISBN 978 0 85725 315 6
What is Nursing? Exploring Theory and Practice (2nd. ed.)	ISBN 978 0 85725 445 0

Personal and professional learning skills titles:

Series editors: Dr Mooi Standing, Principal Lecturer/Enterprise Quality Manager in the Department of Nursing and Applied Clinical Studies, Canterbury Christ Church University and Dr Shirley Bach, Head of the School of Nursing and Midwifery at the University of Brighton

Clinical Judgement and Decision Making in Nursing	ISBN 978 1 84445 468 6
Critical Thinking and Writing for Nursing Students	ISBN 978 1 84445 366 5
Evidence-based Practice in Nursing	ISBN 978 1 84445 369 6
Information Skills for Nursing Students	ISBN 978 1 84445 381 8
Reflective Practice in Nursing	ISBN 978 1 84445 371 9
Succeeding in Research Project Plans and Literature Reviews for Nursing Students	ISBN 978 0 85725 264 7
Successful Professional Portfolios for Nursing Students	ISBN 978 0 85725 457 3
Understanding Research for Nursing Students	ISBN 978 1 84445 368 9

To order, contact our distributor: BEBC Distribution, Albion Close, Parkstone, Poole, BH12 3LL. Telephone: 0845 230 9000, email: learningmatters@bebc.co.uk. You can also find more information on each of these titles and our other learning resources at **www.learning matters.co.uk**. Many of these titles are also available in various e-book formats, please visit our website for more information.

Nursing in Partnership with Patients and Carers

Audrey Reed

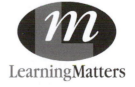

LearningMatters

First published in 2011 by Learning Matters Ltd

British Library Cataloguing in Publication Data
A CIP record for this book is available from the British Library

ISBN: 978 0 85725 307 1

This book is also available in the following ebook formats:
Adobe ebook: 978 0 85725 309 5
ePUB ebook: 978 0 85725 308 8
Kindle: 978 0 85725 310 1

Cover and text design by Toucan Design
Project management by Diana Chambers
Typeset by Kelly Winter
Printed and bound in Great Britain by Short Run Press Ltd, Exeter, Devon

Learning Matters Ltd
20 Cathedral Yard
Exeter EX1 1HB
Tel: 01392 215560
E-mail: info@learningmatters.co.uk
www.learningmatters.co.uk

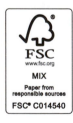

FSC
www.fsc.org
MIX
Paper from
responsible sources
FSC® C014540

Contents

Foreword

There has been a distinctive shift in nursing care from a professionally determined, paternalistic approach towards a more facilitative, partnership approach that respects patients' and carers' needs and wishes. Taking account of the patient's perspective on the nursing care they would like to receive would seem to be an obvious facet of providing sensitive nursing care. The NMC considers that engaging with patients in a partnership over their care is central to nursing. Yet undertaking a partnership approach is not always easily managed; the pressures of busy working environments can drive decision-making, making it hard to fully involve patients or their carers in decisions. Audrey Reed believes that, rather than feeling threatened by carers, nurses should work with them as partners in care and this philosophy pervades the text.

The rationale for a more participatory approach to care is explored by examining the historical background of nursing care and policy drivers. This provides the evidence for this approach to care and equips you with an informed understanding of the more recent, and ground-breaking, development of patient and carer participation in research studies.

Improving individualised patient care is a focal aim of the text. To do this, the factors that may enhance or impede the development of a therapeutic nurse–patient relationship are examined. As this is a complex area, there is help to develop the skills of enabling patients and carers within this relationship to be involved in the decisions made about care.

Many situations in healthcare involve carers as well as patients. Consequently, it is important for nurses to have an insight into the reality of being a carer so they can have effective partnerships with carers and achieve improvements in care. As well as the carer's perspective, family-centred care is explored, helping readers understand the patient's personal support frameworks and how the health issues of one member of a family may affect the rest. Techniques are examined, such as narratives and life stories, to draw out different perspectives on health matters.

An element of partnership care is promoting self-care which requires high quality health information for patients and carers. In this text you will have the opportunity to design health information media to meet these needs. Finally, Audrey encourages you to consider what skills you need to evaluate partnership care and this includes how you may obtain patient and carer feedback.

In each chapter the relevant NMC Standards of Proficiency and NMC Essential Skills Clusters are stated and will be a feature of the Transforming Nursing series.

Shirley Bach
Series Editor

About the authors

Audrey Reed has recently retired from the role of programme manager and nursing lecturer at the University of Leeds. She had been in this role for ten years, during which she had led on curriculum development, including development of a new module on service user and carer perspectives which she created jointly with an 'expert patient'. She has 25 years' experience of teaching, both pre- and post-registration students.

Melanie A. Robbins (author of Chapter 5: Family-centered care) manages the BSc (Hons) Nursing (Child) degree programme at the University of Leeds, with specific responsibility for practice placements. Melanie trained as a RGN/RSCN in Manchester. She worked in children's general and orthopaedic surgery before undertaking a BSc (Hons) Community Nursing at Kings College, London. She worked as a Health Visitor before moving into nurse education.

Acknowledgements

The author would like to thank the following for their help and support in the compilation of this book: Gillian Johnson, formerly University of Leeds, Councillor Eleanor Jackson, Kausar Iqbal, David Proudlove and Valerie Hewison, Carers Leeds.

Also, thanks to all the patients and carers from whom I have learnt so much during my career.

I am also grateful to Dr Felicity Astin, Project Lead, School of Healthcare, University of Leeds, UK (F.Astin@leeds.ac.uk), for the research abstract on page 136.

My thanks also go to: Emerald Group Publishing Ltd for permission to reproduce material (on page 134) from Entwistle, VA, Watt, IS and Sowden, AJ (1997) Information to facilitate patient involvement in decision-making. *British Journal of Clinical Governance*, 2(3): 69–72; and the Royal College of Nursing for permission to reproduce the excerpt on page 96 from *Changing Patients' Worlds through Nursing Practice Expertise: A Royal College of Nursing research report, 1998–2004* (Manley et al., 2005).

Introduction

Over the last couple of decades society has changed so that most people no longer want to be passive recipients of care. The rise in consumerism and the information technology explosion have altered perspectives: people enter healthcare in a different way. Nursing has also changed, and acknowledges and promotes the participation of patients and their carers. This book aims to help every nurse to promote partnership with patients and carers, based on the essential nurse–patient relationship.

Who is this book for?

This book is designed for all pre-registration nursing students. It is not field-specific as patient and carer needs occur in all fields of nursing. An awareness of these needs is also an NMC/EC requirement for adult nurses. There are about six million unpaid carers in the UK and this book will help you to appreciate their needs and how you can promote their involvement in care. Registered nurses will also find here valuable information on involvement policy, the production of health information, and quality assurance, as well as how patient and carer partnerships are fostered.

Why 'Nursing in partnership with patients and carers'?

Partnership is a key theme of current government policy. According to this policy, the perspectives of patients and carers must be sought on care and service provision. Engaging with patients and carers as partners is also central to the NMC *Standards for Pre-registration Nursing* and is, therefore, an essential skill that student nurses must develop. Carers report that their role can be overlooked, but their views and their contribution to care are central to the delivery of high-quality care.

A note on terminology: the word 'patient' has been used to cover all terms for a person receiving care because this is the most widely used term and is used in the NHS Constitution. The use of this term will be explored in the first chapter.

Book structure

Chapter 1 examines how nursing has changed over the last 30 years, from having a paternalistic approach – where the professional is in charge and makes all the decisions – to a facilitative approach through the use of the nursing process. A nursing process approach is about mutuality of purpose and shared decision-making. Developing a therapeutic nurse–patient relationship is central to delivering care in this manner. The chapter will discuss factors that promote and hinder the formation of such relationships.

Chapter 2 sets the context for partnership by exploring current government policy on patient and carer involvement and the NHS Constitution. There is also discussion of patient and carer participation in research studies, as co-researchers as opposed to subjects. The chapter then goes on to explore why patients and carers need to be involved in nurse education, and discusses their role in enabling nursing students to engage with them as partners in care. The chapter concludes by looking at differing levels of participation and the corresponding roles of healthcare professionals.

In Chapter 3 we look at how nursing students need to develop skills of enabling patients and carers. Initially, it is through a one-to-one, nurse and patient and/or carer encounter that partnership is fostered. Only when nurses become more senior will they be concerned with involving patients in service provision decisions. Thus, the focus is on providing individualised patient care and examining the factors that may enhance or impede the development of a therapeutic nurse–patient relationship. Patients and carers will want differing levels of involvement and not all will want to be active participants. Nurses need to assess, therefore, their desired level of involvement in care decisions.

Chapter 4 focuses on carers, their role and their needs. It discusses how their contribution is vital in supporting patients. They are the ones who provide care continuously, and before and after discharge from care services. By knowing the patient so well, they have much knowledge to share, which should be valued and acknowledged. The chapter gives an insight into the reality of being a carer and shows how nurses can best support carers in this role. Rather than feeling threatened by carers, nurses should work with them as partners in care.

Family-centred care is the concern of Chapter 5. It develops the ideas of Chapter 4 in discussing how, in delivering care, you need to understand the patient's personal support framework and how the health issues of one member of a family may affect the rest. The meaning of family and its structure will be examined. Child protection is an issue for all fields of nursing and issues of safeguarding vulnerable adults will also be explored.

Chapter 6 will help you to develop the skills of understanding patients and carers, and will help you to realise the importance of *knowing* the patient and their life story. It therefore looks at a biographical approach to understanding this, and goes on to discuss assessment, which is essential to developing partnerships, as this phase of the nursing process begins the nurse–patient relationship. Good assessment is key to delivering high-quality nursing care and establishing the appropriate level of patient and carer participation.

The concept of self-care is explored in Chapter 7. Promoting self-care is a key tenet of government health policy and is seen by some as essential if the NHS is to remain financially viable – carers are estimated to save the NHS £87 billion annually. Therefore, we discuss how you can promote self-care with patients and carers. The chapter will conclude with an exploration of the roles of self-help groups and the Expert Patients Programme.

Chapter 8 looks at the provision of high-quality health information for patients and carers. In order to be involved in their care, patients and carers must have access to comprehensive and comprehensible information. You will be encouraged to think about how this is designed, produced and distributed. You will have the opportunity to design some information using the Department of Health Toolkit (DH, 2003b). The advantages and disadvantages of different media will also be discussed.

Chapter 9 discusses quality issues. It starts by describing evaluation as the final stage of the nursing process and how this is achieved. It encourages you to consider what skills you need to evaluate care and also how you may obtain patient and carer feedback. It then goes on to explore government policy, the Patient Advisory and Liaison Service (PALS) and quality assurance. You will have the opportunity to think about how these quality issues could be implemented in your practice.

Requirements for the NMC *Standards for Pre-registration Nursing Education* and the Essential Skills Clusters

The Nursing and Midwifery Council (NMC) has established standards of competence to be met by applicants to different parts of the register, and these are the standards it considers necessary for safe and effective practice. In addition to the competencies, the NMC has set out specific skills that nursing students must be able to perform at various points of an education programme. These are known as Essential Skills Clusters (ESCs). This book is structured so that it will help you to understand and meet the competencies and ESCs required for entry to the NMC register. The relevant competencies and ESCs are presented at the start of each chapter so that you can clearly see which ones the chapter addresses. There are *generic standards* that all nursing students irrespective of their field must achieve, and *field-specific standards* relating to each field of nursing: mental health, children's, learning disability and adult nursing. All chapters have generic standards and essential skills.

This book includes the latest standards for 2010 onwards, taken from *Standards for Pre-registration Nursing Education* (NMC, 2010a).

Learning features

Throughout the book you will find activities in the text that will help you to make sense of, and learn about, the material being presented by the author. These activities are designed to help you make sense of the theory discussed and integrate key concepts within your practice. This will be achieved by a variety of activities that will enable you to develop a range of skills. Most activities you can do on your own, but some will require a friend and others you may wish to discuss with your mentor. Some activities ask you to reflect on aspects of practice, or your experience of it, or the people or situations you encounter. *Reflection* is an essential skill in nursing, and it helps you to understand the world around you and often to identify how things might be improved. Other activities will help you develop key skills such as your ability to *think critically* about a topic in order to challenge received wisdom, or your ability to *research a topic and find appropriate information and evidence*, and to be able to *make decisions* using that evidence in situations that are often difficult and time-pressured. Finally, *communication* and *working as part of a team* are core to all nursing practice, and some activities will ask you to carry out group activities or think about your communication skills to help develop these.

All the activities require you to take a break from reading the text, think through the issues presented and carry out some independent study, possibly using the internet. Where appropriate, there are sample answers presented at the end of each chapter, and these will help you to understand more fully your own reflections and independent study. Remember, academic study will always require independent work; attending lectures will never be enough to be successful on your programme, and these activities will help to deepen your knowledge and understanding of the issues under scrutiny and give you practice at working on your own.

Please note that this book is written in an interactive style which is designed to help you with your clinical practice, but for academic work you will need to discuss academic writing style with your tutor.

You might want to think about completing these activities as part of your personal development plan (PDP) or portfolio. After completing the activity, write it up in your PDP or portfolio in a section devoted to that particular skill, then look back over time to see how far you have developed. You can also identify two learning points for each chapter and try to incorporate these in your future clinical practice. You can also do more of the activities for a key skill that you have identified a weakness in, which will help build your skill and confidence in this area.

Chapter 1
The nurse–patient relationship

continued . . . .

By entry to the register:

12. Recognises and acts to overcome barriers in developing effective relationships with service users and carers.

13. Initiates, maintains and closes professional relationships with service users and carers.

2. People can trust the newly registered graduate nurse to engage in person centred care empowering people to make choices about how their needs are met when they are unable to meet them for themselves.

By the second progression point:

3. Determines people's preferences to maximise comfort and dignity.

By entry to the register:

8. Is sensitive and empowers people to meet their own needs and make choices and considers with the person and their carer(s) their capability to care.

3. People can trust the newly registered graduate nurse to respect them as individuals and strive to help them preserve their dignity at all times.

By the first progression point:

2. Engages with people in a way that ensures dignity is maintained through making appropriate use of the environment, self and skills and adopting an appropriate attitude.

By entry to the register:

5. Is proactive in promoting and maintaining dignity.

Chapter aims

By the end of this chapter, you should be able to:

* discuss the implications of using a biomedical model for nursing care delivery;
* identify the importance of respecting patient individuality and promoting dignity;
* discuss the values that underpin patient participation in their care;
* debate issues of power and control within the nurse–patient relationship;
* appreciate the centrality of the nurse–patient relationship in promoting participation.

Introduction

The power to heal lies within the patient and not the nurse.
(Pearson, 1989, p141)

In this quotation, Pearson points to the natural ability of human beings to heal, given the right care. Nursing these days is very much about giving people in need of care the power to control their own care. In fact, encouraging patients to participate in care is now at the forefront of the health agenda in this country. People are no longer expecting to be passive recipients of care, but are being encouraged to actively participate. There is even a new word, 'experience', which acknowledges patients' expertise and their lived experience (Warne and McAndrew, 2007).

Case study

Marie is a 36-year-old secretary who was diagnosed with multiple sclerosis six years ago. On a recent clinic visit, she mentioned to the nurse that she was experiencing increased urinary symptoms, which were seriously impacting on her quality of life. She was finding the incontinence made her working life difficult and embarrassing. The nurse listened to her problems and suggested that she might like to learn to self-catheterise. Marie was hesitant at first because she did not think that she could manage this. However, having discussed it with the nurse and taken the literature she was offered, she said that she would think about it. Marie decided to 'give it a go' and, with the guidance and support of the nurse, successfully learnt this procedure, which transformed the quality of her life.

This case study demonstrates what a difference involving patients in their care can make. This chapter intends to look at how nursing care has changed so as to make this kind of participation easier; it will challenge you to recognise the patient's perspective and participation in care. We will first look at the nurse–patient relationship in the early days of nursing, and then move on to the nursing process and how care is delivered today. Then you are asked to consider the importance of the nurse–patient relationship and factors that may impact on it. The chapter ends by identifying power issues within the relationship and how you as a nurse can empower patients to participate in their care.

The nurse–patient relationship and the biomedical model

In this section, we will consider past influences on the nurse–patient relationship so that you can understand the evolution and importance of patient involvement in care today. Although Florence Nightingale suggested that the role of nursing was to nurture the patient's inner resources and *to put him [sic] in the best state for nature to work on him* (Nightingale, 1859, p133), nursing in the early part of the twentieth century was viewed as a skilled adjunct of medicine, and involved carrying out medical orders. The nurse monitored the effects of these treatments and reported back on the results. It was mechanistic and reductionist, and viewed patients in terms of biological systems and their medical diagnosis. Nurses were not required to make decisions about their care as they were carrying out medical orders. This type of care became known as the 'biomedical model' because it focused on patient diagnosis and pathology. The body was viewed as being made up of biological systems that could be viewed independently of each other. The biomedical model was the standard model of care in the Western world from the early twentieth century right through to the 1970s. Activity 1.1 will help you think about some of the real effects on patient care of using the biomedical model.

Activity 1.1   *Reflection*

- What knowledge would you need to nurse according to this biomedical model?
- What would be the advantages and disadvantages of employing a medical model of nursing care?

An outline answer is given at the end of the chapter.

If you nurse according to a biomedical model of care, the content of your nurse training programme would focus on the biological sciences, pharmacy, carrying out prescribed procedures and making observations. It would not include the social sciences that are in your present curriculum and there would be no interpersonal skills teaching. The nursing component would be about procedures as defined by the hospital procedure manual. This was certainly the case in previous nursing practice (Ford and Walsh, 1994). Nurses were not seen as needing a university education as they were only following orders (Dingwall et al., 1991).

The main disadvantage of the biomedical model is that the human side of care may be neglected (Pearson et al., 2005). Patients may be labelled according to their diagnosis, with people being described as 'schizophrenics' or 'diabetics', which depersonalises them. Being treated as an object like this causes patients anxiety; this form of labelling can all too easily lead to a *type of non-person treatment* (Morrison, 1994, p63). The biomedical model also values high technology, which is associated with scientific development, so low-tech specialities such as care of the elderly have lower status and receive less funding. In this model, the doctor is the head of the team and the person who allows access to the patient. This model did not allow for understanding the person as a whole, which is vital, especially in caring for people with mental illness (Mason and Whitehead, 2003). Finally, because all the information and decision-making rests with the medical staff, patients are precluded from being involved in their own care management and may well be deprived of all the information they need (Pearson et al., 2005).

> ## Case study
>
> *Mrs Smith was an 80-year-old lady who had been admitted for treatment for her leg ulcers. The nurses were always very kind and dressed her legs carefully, but Mrs Smith was sure the dressings smelled and she did not want to mix with the other patients because of this. However, as the nurses only seemed to have time for doing her dressings, she did not like to raise the subject. She became quiet and withdrawn. Also, she lost her appetite and did not eat much, which had an impact on her wound healing.*

The above case study illustrates the problems that may arise with only directing nursing towards the patient's diagnosis. This may seem a strange way of nursing to you, but think about when you have been in clinical practice, as you may find vestiges of this model still around. Have you heard of patients being referred to by their medical diagnosis or bed number, such as 'the appendix in bed 2'? Reflect on your own practice, as it is easy to let language like this slip into your vocabulary; how would you feel if you or a relative were described in this manner? If only the condition is considered, a patient's care may be compromised.

Task allocation

How care is organised and delivered also impacts on the nurse–patient relationship. Just as the *model* of care did not lend itself to patient participation in the past, neither did the *system* of care delivery. The predominant system used was task allocation. A nurse on a ward takes responsibility for a specific task or tasks and performs this task for all patients who require it. For example, for each nurse on the shift, a task would be identified such as 'baths and bedbaths'. She or he would then be responsible for doing all the baths and bedbaths and nothing else for the patients. Pearson (1989) stated that this was the most widespread form of care organisation up until the 1970s, but it continued to exist after other forms of care delivery were introduced. Think about areas where you have worked – do nurses still talk about 'doing the obs' and medicine rounds? Under this system, many nurses may be involved in the care of a patient. This meant that nurses were focused on their task and had little time to build up a relationship with the patient. Tasks are physically orientated, which means that a patient's mental well-being is not addressed. Think about the use of task allocation in the following case study.

> ## Case study
>
> *Josie was an 18-year-old girl who had learning disabilities and difficulties with communication. She was admitted to hospital with acute appendicitis, for which she had surgery soon after admission. Josie was accompanied by her mother and, during the pre-operative phase, she was able to ensure that Josie's needs were understood. However, when she visited Josie post-operatively, she was concerned at how anxious and withdrawn Josie had become. She wanted to talk to the nurses about this, but each nurse seemed to come and carry out a specific aspect of care – one nurse would take her observations, another nurse monitored her*
>
> *continued overleaf . . .*

continued . . .

> *intravenous infusion, another helped her to the toilet, while another nurse gave her antibiotics. All seemed very preoccupied with the aspect of care they were responsible for and did not seem to have time to listen to Josie's mother's concerns nor her suggestions for improving communication. Her mother also found that the teddy that was Josie's comforter was sometimes tucked away in the locker. Whenever she mentioned her concerns to a nurse attending to an aspect of Josie's care, the nurse would reply that he or she was only responsible for that particular aspect.*

This case study demonstrates how the nurses were focused on the allocated tasks and did not appreciate the concerns of Josie's mother. One of the criticisms of task allocation is that no nurse was allocated to look after the emotional needs of patients and carers.

Hierarchies

The above case study shows how the nurses were only focused on their allocated task and did not see the whole picture. The system of task allocation led to the creation of a 'hierarchy of tasks' in which the most technical and closest to medicine were the most valued, and fundamental tasks such as fluids and hygiene were seen as the least important (Pearson and Vaughn, 1986). More recently, however, these latter aspects of care were viewed as so important that the Department of Health created standards for benchmarking these in *Essence of Care* (DH, 2010a). You may also have noted that concerns of relatives reflect these benchmarks. For example, the family appraises the care given to their elderly relative by asking: Is he clean and shaved? Is he wearing his dentures? Has he had a drink?

The system of task allocation supported the existing hierarchical structure of nursing. If you talk to people who were nursing in the 1960s and 1970s, they will tell you how the student nurse on her first ward would hardly dare to speak to a more senior student, let alone the ward sister. The patient, with less power than even the first-year student nurse, therefore found him- or herself very much at the bottom of the hierarchy.

However, in the 1970s there was a growing dissatisfaction with the biomedical model. Trends in society, such as increased consumer expectations and higher health costs, put pressure on nursing to change (Murray and Atkinson, 2000). At this time there was an increase in societal expectations of quality in healthcare and this also drove these changes. The nursing, too, wanted professional status and greater autonomy from the medical profession. Nursing process was seen as a way in which nurses could articulate what nursing contributed to care and take responsibility for their actions.

As a result of these factors, a new model of nursing emerged, based on what became known as the 'nursing process'. The nursing process was first defined by American Ida Jean Orlando in 1961, but appeared in the UK in the 1970s. It was adopted by the General Nursing Council (GNC) as the preferred vehicle for the delivery of nursing care in 1977 (Hogston and Simpson, 2007). We will now look in more depth at the nursing process and how it enabled the development of patient-centred care.

The nursing process and patient-centred care

Activity 1.2   *Decision-making*

- Identify the stages of the nursing process and the skills you need to deliver each stage.
- For each stage, identify what factors will promote or hinder patient and carer participation.
- What do you think are the main underpinning values of the nursing process?

An outline answer is given at the end of the chapter.

In carrying out Activity 1.2, you may have come to realise that the nursing process is more than just making care plans. The nursing process shifts the focus of care away from the task towards the patient, demanding that the whole patient is considered as a person and not as a collection of tasks that require completion. It is a *way of thinking about nursing* (Walsh, 1998, p47) that is person-centred rather than disease-focused. This person-centred approach should also encompass family and carers. Another way of looking at the nursing process is as a way of individualising nursing (Roper et al., 2000). So, with the introduction of the nursing process as the preferred model for nursing care in 1977, nursing moved towards acknowledging the patient as an individual and also making their role in care delivery more active. However, despite the introduction of this system of individualised care being authorised by the GNC, it was not universally accepted by nurses as a way of organising care. This may have been because the nursing process was misunderstood by these nurses, who equated it with the creation of care plans and other documentation, rather than with its underpinning values (Marks-Maran, 1992). In other words, the nursing process was just viewed as a new form of documentation and nothing to do with individualising care and involving patients in decision-making. These essential underpinning values are holistic care, individualised care and the *rights of patients to be treated as unique and autonomous individuals* (Marks-Maran, 1992, p94). These ideas were part of a movement in nursing away from care and care decision-making being just task-orientated, towards becoming dynamic processes based on the nurse–patient relationship. This required a paradigmatic shift from *taking control of patients (taking care of patients) to one of partnership (caring about patients)* (Marks-Maran, 1992, p100).

Case study

In 1993, Beverley Allitt was working on ward 4 at Grantham and Keveseven Hospital. Over a 56-day period, she attacked 13 children, killing four of them and leaving some of the rest with permanent injury. At and after her trial, the press called her the 'Angel of Death'. She was given a life sentence and sent to Rampton

continued overleaf . . .

continued . . .

> *High Security Hospital. An inquiry, which resulted in the Clothier Report (Clothier et al., 2004), was set up into how this could have happened. The main finding was that the healthcare professionals involved could not believe that a nurse would be capable of this behaviour. However, there were also issues of poor documentation and use of the nursing process.*

The Allitt case demonstrates what can happen when nursing care is not documented through the nursing process and care is not, therefore, evaluated. One finding of the Clothier Report was that nurses lacked an understanding of the nursing process (Hogston and Simpson, 2007).

This section, and in particular Activity 1.2, was designed to make you think about the values you associate with the nursing process, and the importance of patient participation in decision-making about their care. It aims to help you to understand what skills you need to develop to deliver care in this way. The next section will explore this further, by thinking about what is meant by treating patients as individuals.

Individuality

Activity 1.3   *Reflection*

What makes you feel unique?

Consider your individual preferences for carrying out the following activities of daily living:

* personal cleansing and dressing;
* eating and drinking;
* sleeping.

These come from Roper et al.'s (2000) model. You may want to use their influencing factors (physical, psychological, sociocultural, environmental and politico-economic) to aid your thinking (see Roper et al., 2000, p14). Discuss your answers with a few colleagues to see what their preferences would be.

This is for individual reflection and no outline answer is provided.

Activity 1.3 should have started you thinking about your personal identity and how you would feel if nurses did not respect your preferences. This will help you to see the importance of the shift to patient-centred care discussed in the previous section of this chapter. Being treated as an individual is essential for people to feel valued and for them to participate in their care. In their analysis of 75 different aspects of care, Richards and Coulter reported that what was seen as most valuable to patients were *patient–professional interactions, communication and being treated as an individual* (2007, p27). Nurses who see patients as individuals are able to provide nursing care of a higher standard (Kralik et al., 1997). Valuing the patient as an individual means that you must also think about how they see the world and what their perspective is on their health problem. In his reflective model, Johns challenged the nurse to ask him- or herself *who is this person?* and *how must they be feeling?* (1991, p1095). Creating a person-centred care plan that identifies individual preferences is important in all four nursing fields, but an example is offered below for an elderly mentally ill adult. An individualised care plan enables nurses to ensure that an individual's care preferences are respected.

Scenario

Imagine you are working in a nursing home and have to draw up a care plan for Mrs Florence Jones, who is 90 and suffering from Alzheimer's disease. Her confusion means that she has difficulty communicating.

Your aim is to ensure that Mrs Jones eats a diet that meets her daily nutritional requirements.

These are the interventions you propose for the care plan.

1. *Ensure that Mrs Jones's dentures are clean and that she is wearing them.*
2. *Check her hands are clean before her meal.*
3. *Remind her of what meal she is eating.*
4. *Encourage Mrs Jones to sit with other residents at mealtimes.*
5. *If she wanders away from the table, encourage her to take finger food with her.*
6. *If she does not eat her meal, offer a snack or a fluid replacement drink – she likes strawberry-flavoured drinks.*
7. *For food preferences, refer to her assessment.*
8. *Offer a snack of fruit (she likes bananas) in the morning and cake in the afternoon.*
9. *Record on her food chart what she has eaten.*

In this scenario, you have demonstrated how Mrs Jones's individual preferences and needs can be communicated to all staff caring for her by means of a care plan. This is especially useful for staff who do not know Mrs Jones very well. How Mrs Jones is addressed is also important and this also needs to be considered.

Names

If patient perspectives are to be considered and partnership promoted, what term is most appropriate for patients' new role in healthcare? Think about the terms in Activity 1.4 and what impact these might have on how you and other professionals might relate to the individual.

Activity 1.4   *Communication*

Write definitions for the following terms.

- Patient
- Client
- Customer
- Consumer
- Service user

Definitions are given at the end of the chapter.

The word 'patient' is the oldest term, and the fact that the other terms mentioned in the activity have been introduced into healthcare reflects changes in society. There is also an attempt by the medical profession to address the previous imbalance in power in healthcare relationships. One definition of the term 'patient' sees it as *reflecting a belief in the recipient of care as a valued person, receiving a service within which they have at least equal rights and a valued role and status* (Elliot-Cannon, 1990, p82). The term 'patient' is used in this book because, although 'service user' is the more accepted term in mental health and learning disability, most nursing literature uses the term 'patient', as does recent government policy.

What is the nurse–patient relationship?

The last section looked at understanding a patient as an individual. But how can you build on this understanding to develop successful therapeutic relationships? We will now look in more detail at the nurse–patient relationship and how central this is to promoting participation in nursing. In clinical areas where the turnover of patients is rapid, this is even more challenging. One way to approach this as a nurse is to value each person who happens to be a patient, and to see each one as a resource (Barber, 1991). Nursing was described by Peplau as *an interpersonal process which with other processes makes health possible for the individual or community* (1952, p55). Although Peplau had a mental health background, her views on the educational and interpersonal element of nursing tie in with the participation agenda. Another way of looking at the relationship is to concentrate on the empathy between nurse and patient (Barber, 1991), in such a way that the patient can be supported in activities that promote health. Essentially, this means that you must feel valued within the relationship to enable you to participate and contribute to improving your health. The nurse–patient relationship is central to the process of nursing (Pearson, 1989), so, throughout each stage of the nursing process you should use your interpersonal skills to build up a relationship with the patient that demonstrates that you value their input. In particular, you need to make sure that your non-verbal communication is congruent with your verbal communication ('walk the talk').

So, how do you develop the kind of nurse–patient relationship that shows how you value the patient? It starts, as with any other professional relationship, at a fairly superficial level (Stein-Parbury, 2000) and then it is your behaviour that makes the difference to the quality of the relationship that is then formed. In the initial orientation phase of the relationship, the nurse has a 'stranger role' (Peplau, 1952) and to develop the relationship from that of strangers, the nurse has to form a therapeutic relationship that values the patient as a partner in their care. Partnership will be discussed further in Chapter 3.

Remember that initial impressions are important, and how you first greet the patient may impact on the subsequent quality of the relationship formed. Think about whether you always introduce yourself and, if appropriate, do you shake a patient's hand? Shaking hands acknowledges the patient and helps them feel valued. For the patient who feels physically unattractive or who has low self-esteem, this will be a morale boost. We will now look at some of the factors that influence the quality of the nurse–patient relationship, including the use of names, dignity, environment, power and control, and empowerment. Consider the following case study and the feelings it engendered in the carer.

The use of names

Case study

The following example of the importance of names is included in Seeing the Person in the Patient *(Goodrich and Cornwell, 2008). It is an ex-nurse talking about the care of her 87-year-old mother on her admission to hospital following a fall.*

> Significantly, the ambulance crew were the only people in the entire seven weeks who formally introduced themselves and asked what she would like to be called. Thereafter, for the first six weeks of her admission, she was called Elizabeth, which is her first name, which she has never been called in her life, ever. She's only ever been called by her middle name. But the NHS IT system records your name. All her labels were wrong. In spite of the fact that on a daily basis all of us told people caring for her that her name is Margaret, and that is what she likes to be called, if they want to call her by her first name, all of them called her Elizabeth. And that became very significant when she became confused.
> *(Goodrich and Cornwell, 2008, p9)*

During assessment, patients are asked what they want to be called, but they may say they want to be called by their first name to comply with staff expectations. You need to consider whether using first names really does promote equality in the relationship or could it be viewed by elderly patients as too familiar or patronising? They may feel that 'Mr Jones' or 'Mrs Jones' shows them respect or acknowledges that a relationship has to be developed. Equally, a child may feel more comfortable being called by a pet name, which may bear no resemblance to the one recorded on the NHS IT system. If a child or adult cannot say what they prefer, make sure you ask their family or carers.

> ## Activity 1.5   *Reflection*
>
> - Write down what your beliefs and values are about the nurse–patient relationship.
> - Would it make a difference if it were termed the patient–nurse relationship?
> - Think about your recent clinical experience and identify factors that you think influenced the nature of the nurse–patient relationship.
>
> *This is for individual reflection and no outline answer is provided.*

Activity 1.5 was designed to help you to realise how your beliefs and values underpin practice and influence care delivery. You may have thought about values such as honesty, empathy and trust. You may have considered how you view patients and how much you value their contribution. Issues that may influence the nature of the nurse–patient relationship are the continuity and the duration of that relationship, as well as the context, environment and the people involved. It may also have made you think about your personal involvement in the relationship. While this will be explored further in Chapter 3, it is worth noting that patients appraise nurses and like to find out about them as people before doing so professionally (Morse, 1991). In another study, patients described nurses as *being engaged or detached* within their nursing role (Kralik et al., 1997, p399).

Dignity

In Activity 1.5, you may also have identified the importance of maintaining dignity and respect in the formation of a positive nurse–patient relationship. Dignity and respect are the key aspects of care identified in *Essence of Care* (DH, 2010a), and research has shown that respect is also a key theme for their relatives as well as patients themselves (Gallagher and Seedhouse, 2002). The NMC states that nurses should *make the care of people your first concern, treating them as individuals and respecting their dignity* (NMC, 2008a, p2). Recently, the Royal College of Nursing (RCN) launched a campaign for the preservation of dignity. In it, they relate dignity to the way people are treated, which should show respect in a manner that demonstrates the person's value as an individual. Preserving dignity is about promoting an individual's worth and their *innate individuality* (Walsh and Kowanko, 2002, p148).

It is clear that preserving dignity is important, but in practice the issues involved are complex. For instance, there have been recent moves to preserve patients' modesty by introducing a different style of hospital gown, because people feel vulnerable if their bodies are exposed inappropriately. People who feel vulnerable are unlikely to have confidence to participate in their own care. As the RCN (2008) identified, a number of studies have highlighted the need to help people to feel in control by giving information and explanations, along with offering choices and gaining consent in order to preserve dignity.

**Research summary: 'Nurses' and patients' perceptions of dignity'
(Walsh and Kowanko, 2002)**

This was a phenomenological study into the meaning of dignity to nurses and patients. It was designed to find out what people's perceptions were of this concept and the factors influencing their view. Participants were recruited from one hospital by volunteering; five patients and four nurses were interviewed. Themes that emerged from nurses' interviews were privacy of body and space, valuing the patient as a person, giving them time and control, and showing respect. These were similar to those identified by patients, which were being seen as a person, having time, time to decide, being acknowledged, and being shown consideration. The study was conducted in Australia, so there may be cultural implications in the findings.

It can be seen from this study how important the nurse–patient relationship is in preserving dignity. Giving control was another important issue for both parties, as was the environment in which care took place. This environment was both physical, as in the facilities available and how they were used, and emotional, where time was given for the patient to make decisions.

Environment

Another factor that may influence the nurse–patient relationship is the environment in which care takes place. The totality of the institution, whether it is a hospital, clinic or GP practice, has an impact on the individual (Goffman, 1961). These places are unfamiliar and anxiety-provoking. Try to remember how you felt when you first started practice learning experience and how anxious the strange environment made you feel. If you do not feel confident in your environment, it will affect your ability to assert yourself and be active in care discussions. You may have felt more at ease in a certain clinical area and, if so, it would be useful to know why that was. It may have been because the staff were friendly and welcoming and knew something about you before you arrived. You may have found your mentor to be particularly supportive of your learning. Feeling supported enables you to ask questions. It is the same for patients – they need their environment to be supportive in order to participate in their care (Hook, 2006).

Also, you may have noticed how the environment is influenced by the way members of the multi-disciplinary team work together. Good working relationships make for a comfortable environment, whereas tensions in the air make people nervous and edgy. In good working relationships, communication is valued and enough time is allocated for it. Where people feel comfortable and confident in their working situation, the atmosphere is more positive. Relationships between staff and patients are influenced by the environment and the degree of privacy (Jones et al., 1997). When staff lack control over their environment, or time schedule, relationships suffer. Nurses also need to allow enough time to engage in a meaningful way with the patient (Hook, 2006).

Power and control

It is important to realise how vulnerable people feel in a healthcare setting. Some of this may arise from past experiences. You may think that you know how people feel and why they are reacting the way they do, but it is only if you listen to them that you will really understand their perspective. One author has written of the patient experience as being one of *crushing vulnerability*, which was attributed to the nurses having power and control (Morrison, 1994, p25).

Activity 1.6   *Reflection*

The weblinks that follow are to sites that contain real-life stories, from all four fields of nursing and covering a range of health issues. They give insight into how it is to live with a long-term condition or disability. Sometimes, you only see a patient for a short time, but they and their families have to learn to live with the health problem.

- Access one of these websites – **www.healthtalkonline.org** or **www.patients voices.org.uk** – and click on some of the stories.
- Explore the scenarios and choose a narrative from one of these sites that is relevant to your practice.
- What impact did these have on your thoughts and feelings?
- What insights did they provide? Did anything surprise you?
- Does this link with any experiences you have had in your own clinical practice?

As this is based on your own insights, no outline answer is provided.

Patients are more likely to feel in control when they are in their own homes and the nurse is their visitor. If you work or have worked in a community setting, you will appreciate the difference in the power base that this affords, as the nurse has no automatic right of entry into the patient's own home. This is clearly illustrated in the following case study.

Case study

Mrs Jolly was an 89-year-old lady who was being taken on a home visit by the occupational therapist and nurse to assess her ability to cope on discharge. When they arrived at her flat, the nurse wanted to use the toilet and requested permission from Mrs Jolly to do so. Mrs Jolly replied 'Wait a minute' and continued talking to the occupational therapist. The nurse tried again but received a similar response. The third time, she explained that the situation was now quite desperate, to which Mrs Jolly replied, 'Now you know how I feel in hospital when I want to use the commode and you tell me to wait a minute.'

Nurses are also in control when they decide when patients can undertake such activities as going to the dayroom or returning to bed.

Both nurses and patients are aware that the power base in the nurse–patient relationship is unequal (Hewison, 1995) and the nurse's style of communication is very important in the way power and control are exerted over the patient; it may be overt or covert (Stein-Parbury, 2000). An example of overt power is when the nurse issues orders, such as telling a patient to return to bed (Hewison, 1995). Think about how you ask permission of patients to undertake nursing procedures. If you say, 'I have come to take your blood pressure, is that OK?', this is a rhetorical question and you are not really offering a choice to the patient. You may have heard nurses use terms of endearment to patients, such as calling them 'dear', which may have been well meant but may sound patronising to patients. How would it make you feel? Using terms of endearment such as 'poppet' puts the patient in a childlike position (Hewison, 1995). Another way in which nurses maintain control is by the use of ward routines such as having set times for taking a bath or having visitors.

This control over patients is often reinforced by the routinisation of the environment and the unwritten rules of the ward (Stein-Parbury, 2000); patients want to keep to the rules and to *fit in* with these to the extent that they may not try to get involved in their care decisions (Biley, 1992, p418). Remember that it is not only what you say that conveys power and control but also your non-verbal communication. So, try to remember that patients are watching your facial expressions for signs of how their behaviour is perceived.

Nurses may think that they control patients' behaviour because of their professional knowledge and expertise, which could be considered paternalistic. Traditionally, nurses did adopt a paternalistic approach towards patients. Paternalism is when restrictions are imposed on an individual's freedom to select actions, for the good of that individual (Mason and Whitehead, 2003). You may think that, as a nurse, you should take control of a situation for a patient's benefit and that, if you do not, a patient may choose a course of action that you consider would be detrimental to their well-being. Equally, however, it may be that this approach is adopted by the nurse as the easiest option because the patient does not have the freedom to question decisions.

Empowerment

Nurses, therefore, need to empower patients so that they can participate in their own care. The NMC explicitly states this as a requirement in the pre-registration standards. But what is empowerment? It is difficult to define as the word has been widely used with different connotations, but it is related to control, being informed and being able to make decisions (Naidoo and Wills, 2001). A useful definition of empowerment is:

> *a social process of recognising, promoting and enhancing people's abilities to meet their own needs, solve their own problems and mobilise the necessary resources in order to feel in control of their lives.*
> (Gibson, 1991, p359)

So, empowerment is an active process that involves facilitation, provision of information and finding solutions. It is not about simply leaving a patient to care for themselves (Marland and Marland, 2000). Empowerment involves enabling patients to consider options and their consequences in order to make informed choices. You need to be involved with giving them the necessary information so they can do this (information-giving will be discussed in Chapter 8). It does not mean leaving patients to their own devices, which could be even more disempowering.

Activity 1.7   *Communication*

Which of the following statements do you agree with?

- I think of patients as partners.
- I feel able to express my ideas in meetings.
- I think that empowering people is letting them do what they want.
- I really listen to what patients are saying.
- I feel comfortable with not being the one in control.
- I determine a person's ability to make decisions on the basis of their medical diagnosis.
- I think some patients want the nurse to be in control.

This is for individual reflection and no outline answer is provided.

Activity 1.7 is designed to make you consider how comfortable or otherwise you feel with not being in total control and making all the decisions. It also raises the question of whether there are times and situations when patients do not want to participate. This will be discussed further in Chapter 3. It is your own attributes as well as those of the patient that lead to successful empowerment of the patient (Gibson, 1991), which is why you need to consider the answers you gave in Activity 1.7.

But it is not always easy to help empower your patients. For example, as a nurse you may not feel comfortable speaking up in a multi-disciplinary setting (Marland and Marland, 2000); there are power issues among healthcare professionals, and sometimes it's the nurse who needs empowering (Trnobranski, 1994). The way an organisation is structured will affect empowerment: if you do not feel the organisation is supportive of you, you may not feel in a position to empower patients. In some institutions, the medical model is still so deeply rooted that it interferes with nurses' ability to empower patients to take control of their health (Chambers and Thompson, 2008), and these authors advocate the continuing education of nurses in empowering skills.

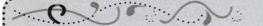

Chapter summary

This chapter has traced changes in nursing and society in order to help you to understand the impact these have had on care delivery, the nurse–patient relationship and patient participation. By appreciating these influences, you should now be able to appraise clinical practice for vestiges of the medical model. Hopefully, you will also have seen a nursing process approach in promoting individuality of care and patient participation. You have been asked to consider the different beliefs and values in nurse–patient relationships and reflect on these in your own practice. Nursing must adopt a facilitative rather than paternalistic approach if participation is to become a reality. Further chapters will pick up the themes explored here to see how to develop these skills further in practice.

Activities: brief outline answers

Activity 1.1 Biomedical model (page 8)

- Knowledge required: anatomy, physiology, biochemistry, pharmacology, pathology, microbiology.
- Advantages: it is cure-orientated, which gives clear direction to everyone, clearly defines the roles of doctor and nurse, and is understood by patients because of its long history.
- Disadvantages: it is reductionist and mechanistic, places an emphasis on medical treatments to the exclusion of alternative therapies, is high value as regards technology and is less appropriate for chronic conditions.

Activity 1.2 Nursing process (page 11)

Stage: Assessment

Skills needed to deliver assessment: observation, measurement and interpersonal skills that include initiating relationships and relationship-building, trust-building and self-disclosure.

Factors that promote or hinder patient and carer participation:

- Promoted by quality of relationship commenced, the participatory nature of the environment, dignity and respect shown, and by appropriate carer involvement.
- Hindered by poor communication, lack of time, and focus on documentation completion.

Stage: Planning

Skills needed to deliver planning: negotiating, prioritising, goal-setting, appraising the evidence base and decision-making.

Factors that promote or hinder patient and carer participation:

- Promoted by acknowledgement and negotiation of their priorities and concerns. Explicit identification of their desired involvement in care. Care extends beyond medical orders.
- Hindered by lack of individualisation of care plan. No identification of variance if care pathways are used.

Stage: Implementation

Skills needed to deliver implementation: clinical skills.

Factors that promote or hinder patient and carer participation:

- Promoted by facilitation and support of patient and carer desired involvement. Interprofessional working.
- Hindered by ignoring preferences of patient and carer. Task allocation.

Stage: Evaluation

Skills needed to deliver evaluation: interpersonal skills, observation and measurement.

Factors that promote or hinder patient and carer participation:

- Promoted by seeking of patient perspective on care outcomes.
- Hindered by only physical criteria being acknowledged.

Underpinning values of nursing process:

You might have mentioned individuality, holism, partnership and the importance of the nurse–patient relationship.

Activity 1.4 Definitions (page 14)

- **Patient**: the word is associated with the patience derived from the Latin word *patiens*, a participle of the verb 'to suffer'. The *Concise Oxford English Dictionary* (2010) definition is *a person receiving or required to receive medical treatment.*

- **Client**: a term that was introduced in the latter part of the twentieth century and used, according to the NMC (2002), to refer to all groups and individuals who have direct or indirect contact with registered nurses and midwives in a professional capacity. Deber et al. (2005) noted that, while 'client' suggests a recipient of professional services, it could also be used for the recipient of the services of a prostitute.

- **Customer**: this term is more suggestive of a market-driven approach, but is rejected by most respondents to a survey by Goodrich and Cornwell with responses such as *Customers is British Rail really* and *Imagine people going into theatre and saying to the surgeon, your next customer's here* (2008, p24). These respondents were from a range of healthcare professionals and patients.

- **Consumer**: Deber et al. (2005) link this with client and customer to note the commercial connotation and the suggestion of market forces.

- **Service user**: Beresford (2005) noted the wide usage of this term, particularly in the fields of mental health and learning disability. He suggested that the term was an attempt to move away from previous labels with negative connotations. However, he also noted that the term 'user' was negatively appraised because of the association with drug users and the implication of manipulation of the individual. Deber et al.'s (2005) study in general care settings found the term 'patient' to be less objectionable, while Sharma et al. (2000) determined that their respondents in a mental health setting showed no universal preference for a particular term.

- **Impact on care**: From these terms you can see a move away from a passive role (e.g. patient) to a more active one, with the use of terms that suggest choice (e.g. user, consumer). Beresford (2005) cautioned that it was all very well employing the acceptable terminology, but more important than language was how people were treated and that this was in an equal rights-based manner.

Further reading

Barber, P (1991) Caring: the nature of a therapeutic relationship, in Perry, A and Jolley, M (eds) *Nursing: A knowledge base for practice.* London: Arnold.

Barber is a nurse educator and psychotherapist who uses reflection to provide an insightful commentary on his hospitalisation following emergency surgery.

Charalambous, L (1992) Write to care. *Nursing Times*, 88(50): 47.

This is a short personal reflection on the value of care planning.

Morrison, P (1994) *Understanding Patients.* London: Bailliere Tindall.

This is a phenomenological study of patients' experiences of hospitalisation.

NHS Executive (1999) *Once A Day.* Available online at www.dh.gov.uk/prod_consum_dh/groups/dh_digitalassets/@dh/@en/documents/digitalasset/dh_4042779.pdf (accessed 6 February 2011).

This is called 'Once a day' because in primary healthcare, on average, practitioners will meet an individual with learning disabilities once a day, and this is an interactive guide to help them meet their needs.

Useful websites

www.dh.gov.uk

This website will give information about government policy on care environments. You can also read about dignity as an *Essence of Care* benchmark, as well as the other identified benchmark aspects of care.

www.rcn.org.uk

This website can be used to learn more about the Dignity in Care campaign and ensuing recommendations for practice.

Chapter 2
Health policy on patient and carer partnership

continued opposite . . .

continued . . . . ●

By the first progression point:

1. Articulates the underpinning values of the *The Code: Standards of conduct, performance and ethics for nurses and midwives* (NMC, 2008a).

By the second progression point:

7. Uses professional support structures to learn from experience and make appropriate judgments.

By entry to the register:

12. Recognises and acts to overcome barriers in developing effective relationships with service users and carers.

Cluster: Organisational aspects of care

14. People can trust the newly registered graduate nurse to be an autonomous and confident member of the multi-disciplinary or multi-agency team and to inspire confidence in others.

By the first progression point:

1. Works within *The Code* (NMC, 2008a) and adheres to the *Guidance on Professional Conduct for Nursing and Midwifery Students* (NMC, 2010b).

By the second progression point:

2. Values others' roles and responsibilities within the team and interacts appropriately.

By entry to the register:

7. Challenges the practice of self and others across the multi-professional team.
10. Works inter-professionally and autonomously as a means of achieving optimum outcomes for people.

Chapter aims

By the end of this chapter, you should be able to:

- discuss health policy that supports patient and carer participation;
- analyse the advantages and disadvantages of Patient's Charters and the NHS Constitution;
- differentiate levels of patient and carer involvement;
- identify forums that promote patient and carer involvement;
- discuss patient and carer involvement in research and nurse education.

Introduction

If you hear me, why aren't you listening?
(Gilbert, 2006, p9)

Gilbert says this is a complaint often made by patients. What do you think it means? Nurses need to understand the difference between just hearing someone and actually listening to them. In the last chapter we looked at how the nursing process promotes shared decision-making, and now we will discuss government policy that is directed at *listening to patients*. This policy is designed to give patients and carers a greater say in the way services are designed and delivered, so that they can become co-producers of care. In this chapter we will also explore how patients and carers can be involved in research and nurse education. Finally, we will discuss differing levels of patient and carer participation, so you can reflect on what this all means for your practice as a nurse.

As we move further into the twenty-first century, all health professionals need to change how they work (Dixon and Dickson, 2008). As a nurse you need to think about helping patients to be active in their care in new and different ways. In the past, people only went to the doctor or saw another healthcare professional when they were ill – nowadays part of every healthcare professional's role is to encourage people to be proactive about their health and engage with new technologies. If you think about it, the old model is no longer fit for purpose: the population is ageing, public expectation for treatment is rising and many people are living with long-term conditions.

In 2002, the Department of Health published the Wanless Report (DH, 2002), which proposed that people need to become more engaged with their health. The idea was that, in doing so, they would make fewer demands on the health service, and save money. This trend has continued, with patients seen as *co-producers of health* (Coulter, 2008, p32), because they had to make decisions about what to do, whether to consult a health professional and, if so, which one. If living with a chronic condition, they had to learn how to cope. What Coulter saw as the patient's key role in producing health was often ignored in health policy, but it was the patients themselves who provided the majority of the care. We need to add carers to this, as we will see in later chapters how they also play a large role in caregiving. We will start exploring this policy by looking at the Patient's Charter.

The Patient's Charter

One of the first steps in the movement away from a paternalistic approach to healthcare towards a patient- and carer-led NHS was the Patient's Charter. Some of you may remember the Patient's Charter being delivered to households throughout the UK, with each home country having its own version. The Charter was established in 1991 and revised in 1995 and 1997. For the first time, it set out a number of rights for patients and carers across a range of services provided by the NHS.

Activity 2.1   *Evidence-based practice and research*

Find and read the original Patient's Charter for your country (the one for England can be found at **www.pfc.org.uk/node/633**).

*   What are the advantages and disadvantages of having a charter of rights?

Access **www.adviceguide.org.UK** and look at the health advice available for your country.

An outline answer is given at the end of the chapter.

You can see if you compare the Patient's Charter with current health advice offered by the Citizens Advice Bureau that the position of the patient and carer has changed during this time. The growth in consumerism in the last 30 years has driven this policy, which seeks to transfer more power to patients and carers and make them central in care provision. The White Paper *Equity and Excellence: Liberating the NHS* sets out the government vision for this and wants patients and carers to have far more influence and choice in the system. *The system will focus on personalised care that reflects individuals' health and care needs, supports carers and encourages strong joint arrangements and local partnerships* (DH, 2010b, p3).

Overview of government policy promoting patient partnership

1997 *The New NHS: Modern, dependable*

The new Labour government sought to respond to changes in society and modernise the NHS. This white paper (DH, 1997) was about promoting integration of care through agencies and organisations working together. There was to be more joined-up practice between health and social care. As well as covering partnership working, it was about patient-centred care.

1998 *A First-class Service: Quality in the new NHS*

The stated aim of this white paper was *the best care for all patients everywhere* (DH, 1998, p3) and set out a ten-year programme. It focused on quality and it was this paper that set up the National Institute for Health and Clinical Excellence (NICE), the Commission for Healthcare and National Surveys of Patient and User Experience. The National Service Frameworks (NSFs) were also established and these made statements of what care patients could expect. Try Activity 2.2 to find out more about a framework in your field.

Activity 2.2   *Evidence-based practice and research*

- Select one of the following, according to your field of nursing:
  - National Service Framework for Older People;
  - Valuing People;
  - National Service Framework for Mental Health;
  - National Service Framework for Children, Young People and Maternity Services.
- Identify issues for patient and carer participation.
- What evidence have you seen in clinical practice of these recommendations being implemented?

This is for individual study and no outline answer is provided.

From undertaking Activity 2.2, you should have found evidence of people working together to promote better health.

1999 *Saving Lives: Our healthier nation*

This white paper (DH, 1999b) sought to promote health by encouraging people to self-manage their own illness, and introduced the Expert Patients Programme (EPP), which will be discussed in Chapter 7.

2000 *The NHS Plan*

The NHS Plan (DH, 2000) set out a vision for services that were designed around the patient and were responsive to them, offering choice and involving them in decision-making and planning. There were to be more non-medical people on boards such as the NHS Modernisation Board and the General Medical Council (GMC). It was about creating a high-quality service with national standards that was available to people and tailored to their individual needs. It proposed better information to inform patient choice. It replaced Community Health Councils, which had existed since 1974 as independent committees representing patient and public interests at local level, with Patient and Public Forums for each Trust. It also established the Independent Complaints Advocacy Service (ICAS) and Patient Advisory and Liaison Service (PALS), which will be discussed in Chapter 9.

2000 *Our National Health: A plan for action, a plan for change*

The Scottish National Executive (2000) produced this report, which was about individuals, groups and communities being able to influence priorities and planning of services with the aim of improving quality.

2001 *Shifting the Balance of Power: Securing delivery*

Notice that title of this white paper again clearly indicated the intention to transfer power to patients and carers. It stated that changes would be delivered in behaviour, culture and processes in order to *put the individual at the heart of everything we do* (DH, 2001b, p2).

The following year another paper was issued that pursued these changes and those of *The NHS Plan*. It was about giving patients greater choice and having a strong clinical focus. It abolished health authorities and prioritised local decision-making.

The Health and Social Care Act 2001

This Act placed a legal duty on NHS organisations to involve and consult patients and the public in the planning and development of services. It formalised many of the proposed changes in *The NHS Plan*. Overview and Scrutiny Committees were also established to watch over and promote health improvements in their areas. They could review any matters relating to the planning, provision and operation of local health services and make reports and recommendations to local NHS bodies, as illustrated in the next case study.

Case study

Eleanor is a member of an Overview and Scrutiny Committee for healthier communities and older people. She has just chaired a panel of councillors to report on whether the changes that the council made to home care services, moving from in-house to commercial provision, had affected the quality of care. In investigating this, the committee researchers spoke to many patients, families and carers. They found a high degree of commitment from both professional and lay carers. The committee did, however, identify problems with parking arrangements in one locality, which resulted in the late arrival of the professional carers. As a result of their report, there were improvements in communication and understanding of the complaints procedure.

2001 *Improving Health in Wales*

This document (National Assembly for Wales, 2001) set out the Welsh strategy, which aimed to promote partnership with citizens and communities in Wales to develop health policy, improve health and reduce the inequalities in health.

2002 The Wanless Report

This report (DH, 2002) set out to assess how the NHS was responding to increased patient and public expectations, technological advances and the changing health needs of the population. It emphasised the importance of better productivity and audit. It recommended the rolling out of the NSFs and their equivalents in the devolved administrations.

2003 The Commission for Patient and Public Involvement

This commission was set up to oversee Patient and Public Forums.

2004 *The NHS Improvement Plan*

This reviewed progress from *The NHS Plan* and declared that the NHS was much more ready now *to ensure that care is much more personal and tailored to the individual* (DH, 2004e, p1). The focus for future developments would be to make them responsive, convenient and personalised for everyone across the NHS. It offered patients choice of healthcare providers and their own HealthSpace on the internet where they could access their care records and record personal preferences. Patient choice was seen as a key driver. There was a requirement for NHS Trusts to seek views on their services and publish an annual report. The EPP was to be rolled out nationally. More emphasis was to be given to prevention and keeping people healthy.

2004 *Securing Health for the Whole Population*

This document (DH, 2004d) recommended developing cost-effectiveness based on public health, and improvements in information delivery. It was felt that both the public and health workforce required more support. Also, there was a reassessment of major health determinants and health inequalities.

2004 *Building on the Best*

This document (DH, 2004b) summarised the findings of the government consultation 'Choice, Equity and Responsiveness'. The main finding was that people wanted services to be shaped around their needs rather than feeling that they had to fit in with the service.

The Commission for Health Improvement was set up to report on whether involvement was having any impact on services. It found that there were many initiatives for patient and public involvement but these were not making real changes to the delivery of care.

2004 *Getting Over the Wall*

This document (DH, 2004c) suggested that patient and public involvement was stuck in the consultation process and was not having a visible impact on patient health outcomes. Therefore, communities needed to have greater say over how resources were spent and patients should have more say in their own care. Patient and public involvement must become an integral part of decision-making, not an 'add on'.

Activity 2.3   *Decision-making*

The *Getting Over the Wall* policy talks about patient and public involvement.

- How are these two types of involvement different?

An outline answer is given at the end of the chapter.

2005 *Now I Feel Tall: What a patient-led NHS feels like*

This document (DH, 2005e) aimed to encourage all managers and NHS staff to appreciate the importance of the emotional elements of patient experience and the relevance of this to creating a patient-led NHS. It was about treating people with dignity and respect, and ensuring a care environment that is safe, comfortable and caring. These issues are discussed in Chapter 1.

2006 *Our Health, Our Care, Our Say*

This white paper (DH, 2006a) followed a widespread consultation and aimed to promote health and social care working together. It offered easier access to services, such as extending GP opening hours, and many health-promotion activities. Also, it extended community services, such as walk-in centres. Information services would be improved.

2006 *A Stronger Local Voice*

This white paper set out government plans for patient and public involvement in health and social care with the aim of building on the existing work of the community and voluntary sectors. This was to be done by building on the role of patient forums by creating Local Involvement Networks (LINks). These would be connected with an area rather than a specific organisation. To find out more, undertake Activity 2.4.

Activity 2.4   *Evidence-based practice and research*

Visit **www.nhs.uk/links** and find out the answers to the following.

1. What is a Local Involvement Network?
2. What powers do LINks have?
3. Who can join a LINk?
4. What services do LINks cover?

Find your local LINk and discover more about what it is doing.

An outline answer is given at the end of the chapter.

LINks, as you can see from Activity 2.4, promote patient and public involvement. The NHS Act passed in 2006 committed health service providers in England to seek this involvement. You can read about how providers should do this in *Real Involvement* (DH, 2008) (see 'Further reading' at the end of the chapter).

2007 *The Health Committee's Report on Patient and Public Involvement in the NHS*

This report (House of Commons, 2007) reviewed progress on patient and public involvement and made 27 recommendations for its future management.

2008 *High Quality Care for All*

This report (Darzi, 2008) supported a tax-funded NHS that was free at the point of need. The continued vision should be about a fair, personalised, effective and safe service – a world-class NHS. The report saw the future as being secured by a focus on prevention, improved quality and innovation to ensure best value for money. Equality should be promoted and discrimination reduced. The quality issues raised in the report will be discussed in Chapter 9. Lord Darzi proposed a new NHS Constitution.

2008 *NHS Choices*

This document (DH, 2008c) set out plans for more comprehensive information services to enable people to make informed decisions about their health and social care. NHS Choices would be a source of personalised digital services. Technology would help to reduce inequalities.

2009 NHS Constitution

This established the principles and values for the NHS in England. Public, patients and staff will be consulted about its renewal, which will be every ten years. The fourth principle clearly states that *NHS services must reflect the needs and preferences of patients, their families and their carers* (DH, 2009a, p3). This is a commitment to all patients and carers being involved in and consulted about care decisions and treatment.

Activity 2.5   *Reflection*

Have you read the NHS Constitution and were you aware of the section on staff responsibilities? (Access it at **www.dh.gov.uk** or **www.nhs.uk**.)

- How do you think having a constitution promotes partnership?
- What do you think about the patient responsibilities outlined in section 2b?

An outline answer is given at the end of the chapter.

2009 *Putting Patients at the Heart of Care*

This white paper (DH, 2009b) clearly spelt out the government's commitment to improving service quality through patient and public engagement and empowerment. The public would be involved in the design and delivery of services. It stated that everyone working in the NHS must participate in this engagement. It also sought to increase the number of people receiving personal budgets, which are direct payments they can use for care.

2010 *Equity and Excellence: Liberating the NHS*

This white paper proposed a *bottom-up* change where services would be determined by front-line staff and patients. This would involve the abolition of Primary Care Trusts (PCTs) and Strategic Health Authorities (SHAs) and devolving their financial planning to general practitioner (GP) consortia. There were also proposals for patients and carers to have more choice of services and more access to information through a range of means. They would also have access to their records and, if they wished, they could share these with third parties such as carers or support groups. Shared decision-making and promotion of partnership were a driving theme, epitomised in the quotation: *no decision about me without me* (DH, 2010, p3).

This white paper also proposed that patients' and carers' views should be represented by a strong independent champion – HealthWatch England. LINks would evolve to become local HealthWatch organisations. The local organisations would then feed information into HealthWatch England, which would be funded by and accountable to local authorities (LAs). It would support people by providing advice on accessing services and making choices about care, as well as providing NHS complaints advocacy.

Government policy on self-care, health information and quality will be discussed in the relevant chapters.

Home countries' policies

Before devolution, policies applied to all home countries, but since then policy is determined by each country. Therefore, if you are in Wales, Scotland or Northern Ireland, you need to visit the websites given at the end of the chapter for the patient experience in Wales, patient and public involvement in Scotland or engagement in Northern Ireland.

An overview of government policy on carers

Carers are included in the NHS Constitution and some of the policy just outlined, but there is also a raft of policy specifically for carers and their welfare. Carers' organisations have played a large part in lobbying for changes in policy, and are continuing to do so. The following is a summary of the relevant policy and law.

1990 The NHS and Community Care Act

This Act placed a duty on LAs to hold consultations with carers when they were determining the services required by the person the carer was looking after. Under this Act, LAs should also consult with voluntary organisations that appear to represent the interests of service users, potential service users or their carers.

1995 The Carers (Recognition and Services) Bill

This bill was significant because it enshrined the concept of 'carer' in law. It also established the right of carers, parent carers and young carers to have an assessment of their own needs. It would assess their ability to provide and to continue to provide care. The results of this assessment must be taken into account by the LA when making decisions about service provision for the person with care needs but, while carers now had the right to an assessment, they did not have rights to services.

1998 The Human Rights Act

This Act gives effect to the fundamental rights and freedoms outlined in the European Convention on Human Rights. These rights focus on matters concerning life and death, and being enshrined in law means that they are rights that government and public authorities such as the NHS must respect. An example of how the right to life might be contravened is when carers put off seeking treatment because of their caring responsibilities.

1999 *National Strategy for Carers*

This strategy (DH, 1999c) had three main strands: information, support and care. Under information, there would be a new charter for carers and quality health information. The NHS Direct helpline would provide carer information. The support strand would entail carers' involvement in planning and providing services, and local caring organisations should be consulted. New powers were to be given to LAs to provide services for carers and the first focus of these was to be about supporting carers to take a break. Funds for this respite were identified and financial support for working carers was to be reviewed.

1999 *Better Care, Higher Standards*

This document (DH, 1999d) set out the responsibility of LAs to create local charters for service users and carers by 2000 so that they would find it easier to access services and be involved in decision-making. These charters were to contain information about local services, standards and targets, local telephone helpline numbers and information about how to complain.

2000 Carers and Disabled Children Act

Under this Act, carers were given rights to packages of assessed support, even when the person they cared for had refused an assessment.

2003 Community Care (Delayed Discharges) Act

Carers were given new rights to services that should be organised before a patient is discharged from hospital. Partnership working between LAs, acute trusts and PCTs was advocated, to ensure that care was delivered in the most appropriate way and to enable a seamless transition from hospital.

2004 Carers (Equal Opportunities) Act

This Act developed a local authority duty to inform carers about their rights to an assessment. It suggested that there should be a strategy for this information to reach *hidden carers*. These are carers not known to the LA. This assessment should include consideration of their leisure, training and work needs or their wish to work. There must be cooperation among LA departments to deal with requests to meet carers' needs.

2006 *Our Health, Our Care, Our Say*

This document (DH, 2006a) set out plans for national information and for a website to be set up by 2009 to enable carers to access sources of support more easily. There would be a training programme, Caring in Confidence, established in 2008. It also announced some funds for emergency care cover and a major review of the 1999 carers' strategy.

2008 *Carers at the Heart of 21st-century Families and Communities*

This white paper was the review of the 1999 *National Strategy Carers* and offered a *transformational New Deal for Carers* (DH, 2008b) with a vision that, over the next ten years, the role of carers should be recognised and valued. Support for them to have a life of their own alongside the caring role and to balance their responsibilities is part of the vision, along with a commitment to address the financial impact of caring. An extra £150 million was identified for PCTs to work with LAs to provide breaks. Pilot schemes were set up to look at such issues as annual health checks for carers and how the NHS might better support carers. Every Jobcentre Plus district will have a Care Partnership Manager who will be able to advise carers about local support services. *Carers will be respected as expert care partners* (DH, 2008b, p7). For young carers, support will be offered to enable achievement of the outcomes in *Every Child Matters* (DCSF, 2003). This was a major policy statement that enshrined the need for authorities to work together to achieve the vision. There was also a commitment to consult carers, their advocates and relevant bodies.

New policy for 2011 and beyond

There is a proposal for a bill to require GPs and health services to identify patients who are carers or who have a carer and take their needs into account. Schools would be required to have a policy to identify young carers. This was in response to research that showed that, if carers were not identified, they were less likely to have a life outside their caring role.

One of the biggest concerns of carers is financial. Carers UK responded to this strategy by highlighting a number of issues, but there is also currently a wider review of benefits being undertaken by the new coalition government. This government has stated that it will refresh the strategy and put an action plan in place for the next five years. Carers' organisations continue to pursue and lobby for carers' interests. Although this legislation and policy exists, carers may have to pursue their case in order to obtain fair treatment. In so doing, they may find other relevant legislation to support their cause, as demonstrated in the following case study.

Case study

A landmark case for carers was that of Sharon Coleman. In 2002, while working as a legal secretary, she gave birth to a son who suffered from breathing problems. Her requests to work flexibly so as better to look after her son were denied and so, in 2005, she took voluntary redundancy but claimed that she was forced to resign because of the unfavourable treatment and harassment. Coleman pursued a claim for constructive dismissal, which was referred to the European Court of Justice. The court upheld the claim, stating that it was discrimination by association. *This could mean that the Disability Discrimination Act 1995 could be used to allow more favourable working practices for carers. Carers UK considered that this could have huge implications for carers who work in the UK.*

Thinking about this case helps you to realise how laws establish rights for carers; but to benefit from these, carers need to know about them and, even then, they may have to struggle to ensure that their rights are upheld.

Have you ever reflected on your own commitment to being involved with the health service, and improving it? You may feel that you have enough on with your nursing education, but try to think of the bigger picture and what you might do in the future. We are all potential users of services, as Bradburn (2003) pointed out, and it might benefit you personally as well as professionally to become involved with one of these organisations or in research.

Patient and carer involvement in research

As a nurse you may have taken part in healthcare research as a subject, or seen patients or carers being subjects, but have you ever thought that patients and carers could be co-researchers? Have you witnessed any studies where this has happened? Involve, the National Advisory Group for supporting public involvement in health and social research, says that this should be an active partnership and that it was *doing with* rather than *doing to* patients (Involve, 2010). UK health policy recommends that patients, public and carers should be involved in all publicly funded health and social care (Smith et al., 2008).

Try Activity 2.6 to explore these issues.

Activity 2.6   *Critical thinking*

For each of the following aspects of research, identify one issue that would need to be addressed for patient and carer participation in healthcare research:

- practical;
- ethical;
- methodological (issues with research process);
- philosophical;
- financial;
- training.

An outline answer is given at the end of the chapter.

Thinking about these issues should help you to realise how important it is that all researchers think about these issues during the planning process. Patients and carers can then receive any necessary training and everyone knows what is expected of them. It is also important to think about how patients and carers can become partners in research studies.

Activity 2.7   *Evidence-based practice and research*

- What do you think patients and carers can undertake in the research process?
- Go to **www.peopleinresearch.org** and watch the video, which will help you to answer the above question.
- How would you feel as a patient about being part of a research team?
- Visit **www.nres.npsa.nhs.uk**, which offers guidance on the requirements for ethical review.

This is for individual study and no outline answer is provided.

Patients and carers are increasingly becoming involved as co-producers in research studies; there is an example of this in Chapter 8, where patients and carers produce a health information DVD. Government policy has also promoted their involvement in the education and training of healthcare professionals over the last decade since *The NHS Plan* (DH, 2000). So, this is the next area we will consider.

Patient and carer participation in nurse education

If patient and carer involvement in care services, as just discussed, is to become a reality, healthcare professionals need to be educated in a way that reflects this philosophy. This is in line with the principles set out in *Shifting the Balance of Power* (DH, 2001b). The NMC standards state that *programme providers must clearly show how users and carers contribute to programme design and delivery* (2010a, R5.1.2). You may be wondering why this needs to be stated, as you meet patients and carers in clinical practice. However, when you meet them in this way, you do not always see the long-term effects of their illness and, also, they may be too ill to tell you how they really feel or be too anxious to do this. For example, a patient who is very depressed may struggle to discuss with you what it is like to live with depression. Also, there remains the power issue, which may impact on our *listening*. You need to learn from patients in situations where they feel free to comment and are not inhibited by the clinical setting (Farrell et al., 2006). Some (e.g. Hasman et al. 2006) believe that nurses and other health professionals need to interact with patient teachers as a part of their training, as the best way to foster and sustain a culture of patient partnership. Just as with research, there are issues to consider with their involvement in education, which Activity 2.8 will help you to understand.

Activity 2.8   *Team working*

Imagine you have been invited to join a curriculum planning group for a new nursing programme at your local university.

* How would you feel?
* What would you want to know?
* Would you be representative?

An outline answer is given at the end of the chapter.

Activity 2.8 raises issues of how you prepare people so they can become involved, and how their involvement is recognised and valued. It can be difficult for a person with a health problem to be the only one on a committee and, also, their health problem could make it difficult to get involved. The following case study demonstrates how patients and carers can be involved throughout the process.

Case study

The university had an involvement advisory group, which was made up of 50 per cent academics and 50 per cent service users and carers. When a volunteer was requested to become a member of a curriculum planning group for the new nursing degree programme, Miriam volunteered. Prior to the first meeting of the group she met with the programme manager, who explained its purpose and what her involvement would mean. She also said to Miriam that she could contact her to discuss any terminology, processes etc. that she was unsure of. Miriam attended the first meeting where she was made welcome and this, together with her preparation, made her feel comfortable to contribute. Her help was enlisted to develop a module on patient and carer involvement.

continued opposite . . .

continued . . .

Miriam identified five issues that she saw as important and these were converted into learning outcomes. Miriam felt fully involved and attended the validation meetings. When the module was delivered, she was part of the module team, which again was 50 per cent academic and 50 per cent patients and carers. It was decided that the module would have some taught content such as a session on the EPP, which Miriam delivered, and a Carers' Awareness day delivered by carers.

Most of the module was delivered by problem-based learning. Each group of students was given a problem that they were then facilitated to research and learn from. The 'problems' were developed from workshops where patients wrote short scenarios of their lives. Students were asked to feed back their findings and the patients attended these presentations, thereby offering their perspective. They also gave written feedback that students could use in their portfolios. Finally, they were asked to evaluate their experience and were paid for their attendance.

Attending the presentations made the students nervous, but it also offered invaluable feedback. A wheelchair service user who had three small children under five was able to point out to the students that they had not considered how she looked after them, nor the impact of her paralysis on her sexuality. Meeting patients and carers in this way, outside a clinical setting, helps you gain a clearer understanding of how their condition affects their daily lives. You may also have noticed in the scenario that the students were given written feedback. This is in line with the latest NMC standards, which state that *programme providers must make it clear how service users and carers contribute to the assessment process* (2010a, R8.1.4). Patients and carers as recipients of nursing are ideally placed to advise on the qualities needed. If you have yourself been a patient or carer, you will appreciate how differently you see things from this perspective as opposed to your professional one.

One project that is examining how patient and carer feedback might be captured is the ALPS (Assessment and Learning in Practice Settings) project. This project among five universities in northern England has developed common competencies for 16 different health and social care professionals. One of their aims is *to develop the tools to enable students to collect a wide range of workplace formative and summative assessments from professional assessors, self, peer and service-user ratings* (Holt et al., 2009, p270). In doing this, they have worked with and incorporated the ideas of service users and carers. You can find out more about the project by visiting **www.alps-cetl.ac.uk**. In your reflective journal, reflect on the contribution that patients and carers make to your curriculum and what you learn from this.

We have seen that government policy is pushing the NHS to involve patients in service provision, research and education. But do people want this sort of involvement and, if they do, to what level? It may not be possible to avoid participating (Perakyla et al., 2007) because, when you enter a healthcare situation, you are already involved. Being actively involved as a patient or carer in service planning, research and education is something different. Participation was seen by Hickey and Kipping (1998) as a continuum, starting with a consumerist approach. Here, people, as consumers, were given information and consulted and could make judgements about the service, but power was with the professional. Moving along the continuum, power was given to the person, involving a democratic approach, which Hickey and Kipping saw as meaning partnership, the ultimate position on the continuum being user control. As you can see in this latter situation, power rests with the patient or carer.

Government policy is seeking to move the NHS towards democratisation. As professionals, nurses have a parallel role in this process. Where you do not involve your patient you can be seen as paternalistic, but when the patient is autonomous you can act as an agent. When both are equally involved, this can be seen as *co-determined involvement* (Thompson, 2007, p5). At this level of participation, self-help and user groups are important (Bradburn, 2003), which we will look at in more detail in Chapter 7.

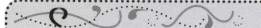

Chapter summary

This chapter has outlined government policy on patient and carer involvement in care and service provision. Just as you have individual preferences for levels of participation, so do patients and carers, which we will explore in the next chapter. In later chapters, we will discuss your responsibility for implementing these policies in practice by enhancing patient and carer self-management, developing high-quality health information and, above all, listening to patients.

Activities: brief outline answers

Activity 2.1 The Patient's Charter (page 27)

Advantages
- Clearly articulates what patients can expect, which represented the first time this had been spelt out.
- Offered opportunity to have information in different languages such as Welsh.
- Set standards against which care could be measured. Commissioners of services could use this.

Disadvantages
- Not legally enforceable and did not give additional legal rights.
- No contractual arrangement with service supplier.
- If it does not happen, patients can only complain.
- NHS staff not consulted in its production.
- Setting target times might mean people with less serious conditions were treated in preference to people with more urgent problems in order to meet targets.
- Unrealistic expectations of patients could be raised.

Activity 2.3 Patient and public involvement (page 31)
- Patients are receiving services and view issues from this perspective.
- The general public have a global view, which may be influenced by different priorities.

Activity 2.4 LINks (page 31)
1. A LINk is a network of local people, groups and organisations in every local authority. LINks were established by the Local Government and Public Involvement in Health Act 2007.
2. LINks have a range of powers, making reports to the Overview and Scrutiny Committees and obtaining responses.

3. Anyone can be part of a LINk. Members include individuals, user-led organisations, and local and voluntary sector organisations.
4. All health and social care services commissioned by the NHS and local authority. Also, independent providers of publicly funded services, but not children's services.

Activity 2.5 NHS Constitution (page 32)
- The Constitution permits values to be clearly stated and shared.
- It empowers patients and staff by stating their rights.
- It strengthens accountability.
- In partnership, both parties have responsibilities and government policy is seeking to outline patients' own responsibility for their health.

Activity 2.6 Aspects of research (page 37)
- Practical: access, mobility, transport and meeting places.
- Ethical: if direct contact with other patients, Criminal Records Bureau (CRB) checks and confidentiality.
- Methodological: lack of knowledge of research process.
- Philosophical: values – what is the value of patient knowledge?
- Financial: expenses, payment of involvement; affects benefit payments.
- Training: how will this be provided?

Activity 2.8 Patient involvement in education (page 38)
- Apprehensive, wondering what is involved, how many people will be at meetings, whether you will understand what is going on, hoping your health problem will not interfere, and so on. Am I being invited as a 'token' to fulfil requirements?
- Where will the meetings be, how long are they, how do I get there, will I be paid and how? Will this affect my benefits?
- How were you selected? Do you know what other patients and carers think?

Further reading

Department of Health (DH) (2008) *Real Involvement: Working with people to improve health services.* London: Department of Health.

This is a comprehensive, managerial guide to all aspects of involvement required under the NHS Act 2006.

Dimond, B (2001) Patients' rights and the Patient's Charter, in *Patients' Rights, Responsibilities and the Nurse.* Salisbury: Mark Allen.

Chapter 7 provides further background information about the Patient's Charter.

Nolan, M, Hanson, E, Grant, G and Keady, J (2007) *User Participation in Health and Social Care Research.* Basingstoke: Open University Press.

The first chapter is about research involvement and the rest of the book has chapters on different research projects in different fields of nursing and also social care in which patients and carers have been involved.

Smith, E, Ross, F, Donovan, S, Manthorpe, J, Brearley, S, Sizia, J and Beresford, P (2008) Service user involvement in nursing, midwifery and health visiting research: a review of the evidence and practice. *International Journal of Nursing Studies*, 45: 298–315.

This paper offers a comprehensive overview of the current position with regard to patient involvement in research and makes suggestions for theory and methods development.

Thompson, A (2007) The meaning of patient involvement and participation in healthcare consultations – a taxonomy, in Collins, S, Britten, N, Ruusuvuori, J and Thompson, A, *Patient Participation in Health Care Consultations.* Basingstoke: Open University Press.

This is a useful discussion of different levels of patient participation.

Useful websites

www.alps-cetl.ac.uk

The Assessment and Learning in Practice Settings project, whose goal is to extend excellence and innovation in assessing practice, helping students to learn both within their professions and across professional boundaries.

www.alps-cetl.ac.uk/essen/player.html

This video clip on the ALPS website discusses guidelines for service user and carer involvement in education. While this is based around involvement in education, much of what is discussed is also relevant for facilitation of patient and carer involvement in research and policy-making.

www.dh.gov.uk

Access this site to find the various Acts outlined in this chapter. (They can also be found at **www.legislation.gov.uk**).

www.engage.hscni.net

Access this site for policy on stakeholder involvement in Northern Ireland.

www.invo.org.uk

Involve promotes public involvement in the NHS, public health and social care research, in order to improve the way research is prioritised, commissioned, undertaken, communicated and used.

www.show.scot.nhs.uk

Click on 'Involvement and Participation' to explore Scottish policy for patient and public involvement in the health services.

www.wales.nhs.uk

Look at this site for policy on delivering the new NHS for Wales and patient experience.

Chapter 3
Patient participation and partnership

continued . . .

By entry to the register:

12. Recognises and acts to overcome barriers in developing effective relationships with patients and clients.

13. Initiates, maintains and closes professional relationships with service users and carers.

2. People can trust the newly registered graduate nurse to engage in person centred care, empowering people to make choices about how their care needs are met when they are unable to meet them for themselves.

By the second progression point:

1. Actively empowers people to be involved in the assessment and care planning process.

5. Provides personalised care or makes provisions for those who are unable to maintain their own activities of living, maintaining dignity at all times.

By entry to the register:

14. Actively helps people to identify and use their strengths to achieve their goals and aspirations.

5. People can trust the newly registered graduate nurse to engage with them in a warm, sensitive and compassionate way.

By the first progression point:

4. Provides person centred care that addresses both physical and emotional needs and preferences.

By entry to the register:

9. Engages with people in the planning and provision of care that recognises personalised needs and provides practical and emotional support.

Chapter aims

By the end of this chapter, you should be able to:

- discuss the meaning of participation and partnership in nursing care;
- analyse factors that influence patient participation and partnership;
- debate the role of handover in promoting patient participation;
- discuss the emotional component of enabling patient participation;
- reflect on developing the skills required in patient participation.

Introduction

In Chapter 2 we looked at the policy that is driving the agenda for patients' participation in their care. This chapter looks at the way we promote patient participation in modern healthcare today, and will focus on how you as a nurse can develop your ability to make patient participation and partnership work. We will look at the meaning of both 'partnership' and 'participation', and what makes them happen – or not – in the delivery of care. The chapter will also look at this from the point of view of patients: what are the advantages and disadvantages to them?

Patient participation

First, we need to decide what we mean by 'patient participation'. It is a complex concept, sometimes used as though it means the same as 'partnership', 'involvement' and 'patient collaboration' (Jewell,1994; Cahill, 1998a). These are similar terms but mean something slightly different. The *Concise Oxford English Dictionary* (2010) notes that 'participation' was derived from the Latin verb *participare*, meaning *share in* and participation was *taking part*. Participation, then, enables a patient to consider different treatment options and decide what is their preferred approach and/or treatment. It gives the patient or carer an active rather than a passive role, unlike in the biomedical model as discussed in Chapter 1. From what has been discussed so far, it might seem that this is the only approach. However, we know that some patients may not want to change. Some elderly patients may be used to a system where the nurse makes the decisions and tells them what to do; participation may be very confusing and a little threatening. The elderly are less likely to want to participate in care and yet, as they have more long-term conditions than younger patients, they would benefit from doing so. Taking part in decision-making is not the easy option. For example, nurse education expects you to be active in your learning and to solve problems, but sometimes you may feel that you just want to sit back and be told; listening to lectures is quite attractive. Reflect on this in Activity 3.1.

Activity 3.1   *Reflection*

Think about a situation in which you have been the recipient of care.

- Were you active or passive in the decisions that were taken?
- Was this your choice?
- What are the advantages and disadvantages of being active or passive in healthcare?

An outline answer to the last question is given at the end of the chapter.

As you can see from Activity 3.1, having a choice makes a difference between being active or passive. In thinking about the advantages, you may have felt more inclined to follow the advice, if this was your choice, and you may have felt that you made quicker progress. However, the disadvantage is that you have to take some responsibility for your actions and not everyone wants to do that.

Self-care

The idea of self-care is not new: it was first introduced into nursing in the USA with the work of Orem (1985), and there has been a growing emphasis on self-care ever since. Coming from the West, it is an idea steeped in Western values, which will not be comfortable for everyone. The UK is a multicultural society, and not all cultures are happy to adopt the idea of self-care. Nurses need to be culturally sensitive, so don't assume that all patients want to self-care. Make sure that you assess each patient as an individual and find out how much they want to participate. (We discussed the importance of individualising nursing care in Chapter 1.) It is important that we find out what people prefer, *and respect individual needs and preferences* (Cahill, 1998a, p358).

Factors influencing participation

We have seen that a patient's age and culture are factors influencing their participation in care, but there are others: the diagnosis, previous experience of healthcare, and educational background. Patients with fewer years of education are less likely to want to participate in care decisions (Smith and Draper, 1994). It is important that you assess each patient and carer individually to find out what level of participation and control they wish to have. Remember that assessment is an ongoing process and people change: they learn and grow and change their minds. When people are first ill, they may need to be passive, but as their health improves they may want to be more involved.

In fact, how ill or well people feel are key factors in their desire to participate. *Being too ill* and *If I am well enough* were two themes identified in research by Biley (1992, p416). If you have been ill yourself, you may have just wanted to be looked after. Patients who are very ill may feel too weak or disorientated to make decisions and, in some cases, patients may be deemed mentally unfit to do so by law.

What about the disadvantages of participating? In Activity 3.1 you may have identified that you did not want to take responsibility, or were worried about doing something wrong. If you are in a strange environment or anxious, you want to conform and avoid mistakes. Patients worry about what they are allowed to do and when. Can they take a bath when they want, and what time do they have to turn their lights out at night? It is important that patients receive information about routines and facilities before they arrive, and frequently during their stay.

Sometimes patients agree to be involved because that is what the nurses expect, and they want to *toe the line* (Waterworth and Luker, 1990, p973). They want to do things right and please the nurse rather than participate. Nurses sometimes forget that patients see us as authority figures (Smith and Draper, 1994) whom they do not want to displease. It is easy to forget, when you are very familiar with an area, how strange it can be when you enter it for the first time. Remember your first practice learning experience? You need to be welcoming, both in your verbal and non-verbal communication – smile, attend and take time. Patients should be participating because they want to and not because they feel they have to.

Another factor in participation is whether patients feel they have enough knowledge: they may see the issue as one needing professional expertise. The theme of *If I know enough* arose in research by Biley (1992, p417), who found that some patients may be more keen to be involved in decision-making about non-technical aspects of care, such as activities of daily living and medication, rather than in technical aspects of treatment, which they preferred to leave to the healthcare professional. Finally, Biley discussed the theme of *If I can* (1992, p418), by which the respondents meant organisational issues, such as the structure of the environment and time constraints on staff. We will look at these two issues later in the chapter.

Defining attributes for participation

Research summary: Cahill's analysis of participation

Jane Cahill's (1998a) research was aimed at discovering the features of 'participation' that define it. To do this 'concept analysis', she undertook an extensive literature review of the subject, and used a recognised analytical framework to identify the defining attributes of the concept. These are her results.

1. *A relationship must exist.*
2. *There must be a narrowing of the appropriate information, knowledge and/or competence gap between the nurse and patient using suitable modalities in different contexts.*
3. *There must be a surrendering of a degree of power or control by the nurse.*
4. *There must be engagement in selective intellectual and/or physical activities during some of the phases of the healthcare process.*
5. *There must be a positive benefit associated with the intellectual and/or physical activity.*

(1998a, p565)

What do these attributes mean in practice? Let's look at an example of how partnership works.

Case study

Kirsty is a 13-year-old girl who suffers from epilepsy. She has regular check-ups at her local hospital, where the paediatrician recommended that she try a ketogenic diet. Kirsty was not too keen on this idea, as she thought she might gain weight, be seen as 'different' and have difficulty when eating at friends' houses. The paediatrician suggested that she and her mother talk this through with the epilepsy nurse specialist, Sue, and the dietitian. Kirsty knew Sue well and listened to what she suggested. Sue gave Kirsty some information about the diet and told her about a blog that had been created about the diet. She offered to talk to her mother about it as well. Kirsty agreed to discuss the diet with the dietitian after she had read all this and the blog entries. Together, they planned the diet for Kirsty, which she found helpful in controlling her seizures.

Can you identify Cahill's defining attributes of partnership from the case study? First, Kirsty had built up a relationship with the epilepsy nurse and it was through this relationship that she agreed to pursue the diet further. Relationships are at the heart of patient participation, so you need to reflect on your ability to develop relationships that are supportive and that encourage the patient to take an active part. You can learn a great deal by watching experienced nurses to see how they use their interpersonal skills to build good relationships with patients and carers.

Cahill's second defining attribute of partnership is about information and how it is given. If there is a knowledge gap between you, as the nurse, and the patient, you need to give necessary information to the patient in the best way for them, which may not be the easiest for you. Here, the nurse used written information that was suitable for Kirsty. She thought about Kirsty's level of education and how best to give information so it would be meaningful for Kirsty. The production of health information will be discussed in more detail in Chapter 8. Kirsty is a teenager and uses social networking sites constantly, so Sue also told Kirsty about a blog called 'Matthew's friends', so that she could find out what people her own age thought about it. Now Kirsty does not always have to be asking what she can or cannot eat. Sue may also use texting to see how Kirsty is getting on.

The third of partnership's defining attributes is about power or control. Sue has to think about Kirsty's relationship with her mother, too, and any power and control issues there. Kirsty's mother saw the importance of Kirsty feeling in control of decisions about her health problem, as she has to live with this; if she agrees to the treatment plan, she is more likely to adhere to it. Besides, many mothers are gatekeepers for the family diet, which is another reason you must include relatives and carers. The school nurse might also be involved and help to support Kirsty in her dietary choices at school. Sue is encouraging Kirsty to make decisions and to feel that she has power over them. Kirsty is a teenager and you may remember that, as a teenager, you did not like being told what to do and would rebel if you felt that you were being dictated to. In nursing we sometimes need to relinquish control, as the nursing role in patient participation must be facilitative rather than controlling or telling.

The fourth defining attribute is about engaging with the process and understanding it. Kirsty read the information and tried to understand the benefits of the new diet and its possible side effects. She appreciated the last attribute, which was that this could benefit her health by improving the control of her seizures.

So, if you think about Cahill's defining attributes of partnership, it will help you remember the ways in which patients are enabled to become involved in their care decisions. Nurses need the ability, the willingness and the resources to enable patients and families to become involved (Stratford, 2003). For this, nurses need:

- *knowledge;*
- *effective communication;*
- *environment;*
- *resources;*
- *attitude.*

(Stratford, 2003, p140)

We will now look at each of these requirements in turn.

Knowledge and communication

In the case study we saw how nurses need to communicate knowledge to the patient, and reduce the difference between their knowledge bases. This works both ways: there will be times when the patient will know more than you. What about your own knowledge base? A helpful tool to use when considering your knowledge base is Barbara Carper's (1978) 'Ways of knowing'.

The first way of knowing is having *empirical knowledge*. This would be your evidence-based, up-to-date knowledge of the subject area. It is important to remember that patients and families have access to a wide array of information including websites, which can have content that is unreliable. You need to have a robust knowledge base so that you can advise patients and families about the quality of information they may have accessed for themselves, making sure you do it in a non-judgemental and balanced way. If they have any hearing or visual difficulties, you need to take that into account when delivering health information. If you do not have the information, you need to be honest and say so, but offer to find out or offer suggestions as to how they can access what they want to know.

Carper's second way of knowing concerns *aesthetic knowledge*. This is the empathetic or artistic side of nursing, including how you come across to patients, and your manner. It is the caring that is conveyed in the way we communicate with patients. Following on from this, the third way of knowing is *self-knowledge*. Self-awareness is an attribute that you need to develop during your training and beyond. Try to seek feedback from your peers and mentors, from people who will offer you supportive and constructive feedback. Ask your colleagues, 'Honestly, what sort of impression do I make?' We are not always aware of how we come across to others. In particular, our non-verbal expressions may be misinterpreted. Also, you need to be aware of how your beliefs and values could influence your actions, and make sure they don't interfere with your caregiving. Nurses must be a *knowing self* and *before we can help others we need to have insight into how we function as a person* (McCormack and McCance, 2006, p475).

Finally, Carper (1978) suggests that we need *ethical knowledge*. You may be studying ethics as part of your course, but here you need to think of that knowledge in the context of such ethical issues as autonomy and informed consent.

You will notice *effective communication* in Stratford's list. Listening is a key skill that is vital in understanding the perspective of patients and carers. You need to hear where they are coming from in order to understand what they want and what they need to know. Try to use open questions and, above all, avoid leading or rhetorical questions. Give them time to answer and do not finish sentences for them, even when they seem hesitant or you are sure you know what they mean. Also, it is useful to reflect back what they have said to check for meaning: 'So, you're saying that you have some doubts about going home?' Remember your non-verbal communication channels and maintain good eye contact; think about your body posture. People who are anxious find it difficult to retain information, so it needs to be repeated and reinforced. This reinforcement may well be in written form and this will be discussed further in Chapter 8.

Environment and resources

The environment is next on Stratford's (2003) list. In Chapter 1, we learned about the importance of the setting in the formation of supportive nurse–patient relationships. These relationships will be difficult to form in an environment of rigid and inflexible routines (McQueen, 2000). Good interdisciplinary working is very helpful in offering a team approach to participation. The environment must be supportive of these working relationships, with sharing of power, and staff should be able to try new ways of doing things (McCormack and McCance, 2006). Try to make the physical environment welcoming and friendly so that patients feel at ease in thinking about what they need. You need to think about creating some privacy for patients and families so they can discuss and consider options; screens do not give real privacy and may prevent patients from saying what they would like to.

Resources will vary but try to be creative with what is available. One resource that is often cited as being in short supply is time. This is a challenge, but examining how care is delivered and reviewing care practices may highlight areas where time could be saved. It is difficult when you first start carrying out nursing activities to do anything other than concentrate entirely on what you are doing, but as you become more experienced and competent you will find that you are able to chat while you work. This is why activities such as bathing patients should not be regarded as healthcare assistant work. Giving intimate care to a patient makes you available for them; it is at this time that they may feel more comfortable raising issues with you (Williams, 2001a). Patients, too, perceive time to be in short supply and do not want to waste nursing time.

Attitude

Lastly, Stratford mentions attitude. By this, she means nurses' attitudes to patients participating and how willing nurses are to relinquish power. Again, the issue of control arises and, with this, their willingness to acknowledge patients' expertise and knowledge of their own condition. You need to develop the skills of enabling and speaking up for patients, when they agree for you to do this and feel unable to do so themselves. In doing this, you may feel that you are developing a partnership with the patient. It seems that we need participation first, before we develop a partnership (Cahill, 1998b). In the next section we will look at the meaning of partnership.

What is partnership?

One of the six key themes in the RCN (2006) definition of nursing is partnership; that shows how important it is. Partnership means different things to different people and may vary according to the context. One definition of partnership is *an association between nurse and patient where each one is a respected, autonomous individual with something to contribute to a joint venture and in which both work towards an agreed goal* (McQueen, 2000, p726). Here, partnership is about a close association that is formed for the purposes of meeting an agreed target. People disagree as to whether there needs to be equality between the parties; some say this is unattainable – just an ideal. It could be argued that patient and nurse will never be equal because the nurse has access to resources that the patient may need but can only access with the nurse's help. Before considering this in more detail, you may find it useful to consider what you think and know about partnership already. Activity 3.2 is designed to help you to do this.

Activity 3.2   *Team working*

- What types of partnership can you think of?
- What attributes make for a good partnership?
- What skills do you have and what do you need to acquire to develop a working partnership?

An outline answer is given at the end of the chapter.

Activity 3.2 should have made you think about what constitutes a partnership. Some people think about partnership in terms of its attributes rather than giving it a simple definition (Hook, 2006), and this may be helpful in thinking about what you need to develop in practice to maintain good partnerships. These same attributes will also be useful when working as part of the multi-disciplinary team.

The attributes identified by Hook are *relationship, shared power, shared decision-making* and *patient autonomy* (2006, p133). Yet again, you will see how the nature and quality of the relationship the nurse has with the patient is central to achieving partnership and participation. It is not enough for there just to be a relationship between the nurse and patient; it needs to be developed through the process of that relationship, which is *the specific way in which the health provider and client work and interact together* (Gallant et al., 2002, p151). Central to this process are power sharing and negotiation. It is worth remembering the differing knowledge bases of the two participants in the relationship: the patient has a wealth of knowledge about their life and body; the nurse has a professional knowledge of the patient's condition. The process must be about sharing this information to negotiate the best possible outcome. Partnership is about sharing.

However, the patient may not always feel that they are being treated as a partner, particularly when they are relating to more than just the nurse. You need to be aware of the patient's perspective and be supportive of them in expressing their viewpoint. Consider the scenario in Activity 3.3.

Activity 3.3   *Communication*

Imagine that you have, or your child has, complex health needs. You have been invited to attend a meeting with the multi-disciplinary team to discuss these health needs. There will be a number of different professionals there, some of whom you have dealt with before.

- What would be your thoughts and feelings prior to the meeting?
- What would you need to do to prepare yourself for this meeting?

An outline answer is given at the end of the chapter.

If you have managed to see this from the patient's or carer's perspective, you can understand how power differentials exist and how intimidating these can be. It is worse if you do not have the education or knowledge to understand the context or the situation and its potential. You need to understand how vulnerable patients can feel, and how they need to be supported to be able to put their viewpoint across in such situations.

Even in hospital ward rounds, the patient is often numbered and put at a disadvantage by the use of unfamiliar language. This will be discussed in more detail towards the end of the chapter. We saw earlier that, when it comes to participation, not all patients want to share decisions; patients may also struggle with the idea of being partners. This may be because they feel powerless, particularly where parents/carers feel that their caregiving is being scrutinised by professionals. They may worry about what might happen if nurses know intimate family or personal details. To help you think about this, examine the issues in the following case study.

Case study

Julie is an 18-year-old single mother of a two-year-old boy with Down's syndrome. She has little family support and struggles to manage physically, emotionally and financially. You visit her as a health visitor to offer support and advice, but Julie is concerned that you are snooping as she is aware that the neighbours complain about her son's crying. She is unaware of the role of the health visitor.

From this, you can see that a mother, particularly one who lacks family support, may be wary of professional interventions and suspicious about any dealings with nurses. In a study on power and partnership in the field of child surveillance, Wilson (2001) concluded that the two parties need to feel free to be honest with each other. She described the power in such relationships as being in 'ebb and flow'. Honesty is certainly a key component in a partnership; patients may never feel truly that they are partners if nurses cannot be entirely open. Difficulty with being open is just one factor that makes participation and partnership with patients hard to achieve. In the next section we look at some of the others.

Factors inhibiting participation and partnership

Although nursing has embraced the idea of patient participation in recent years, patients may not always see it this way. Many patients want more involvement in care decisions (Richards and Coulter, 2007); in fact, 32 per cent of primary care patients and 48 per cent of hospital patients say they had not been sufficiently involved. In mental health, there is a decline in patient experience of involvement. You should reflect on the reasons for this, as you may find that these occur in your practice.

First, a nurse may think it takes too long to ask patients what they would like to do, and it is quicker to do it yourself. Reflecting on this, you realise that it does take longer sometimes to help a patient to learn, for example, to self-medicate or give themselves an injection. It is tempting to just do it, but who is that benefiting? Taking time to explain and discuss care issues with patients should motivate them and mean that they are more likely to understand what they need to do. This should lead to their having fewer problems in the future, which will *save* time.

Second, a nurse might not ask patients about how they cope with their health problem, because this somehow suggests they lack knowledge and seem unprofessional. Some nurses find it too difficult to accept that they can learn from patients; nurse education should promote learning through reflective and reflexive activity to help nurses cope with this without becoming anxious or resistant (Warne and McAndrew, 2007). As discussed at the beginning of Chapter 1, these authors think that nurses should see the value of patient 'experience' and recognise patients as a valuable source of learning. In other words, instead of feeling threatened by the patient's greater knowledge, you should use it to expand your own.

Throughout your nursing career, you can learn so much by listening to patients and finding out how they cope with their problems. You only have contact with a patient for a relatively short time compared with the time they live with the condition. If you value the patient's perspective and experience, they will not view you as incompetent.

There are still vestiges of the medical model and a paternalistic approach in healthcare. Nurses may be reluctant to share power in decision-making because they feel that they have the professional knowledge and they know best. If you think about this, you may realise that it can be easier and more attractive to make decisions for people. If you stay in control, particularly of information, then patients are not in a position to argue. As already shown, patients have concerns about conforming and not being viewed negatively. Some nurses freely admit to maintaining control by giving only selected information (Henderson, 2003). Patients in that study also reported being persuaded to take certain actions and not having sufficient information to act otherwise.

Emotional labour and nursing intimacy

Another factor that inhibits participation and partnership may be that nurses are still task-orientated and only interact with patients when undertaking the physical care that patients require. Nurses can use task allocation (see pages 9–10) as a defence mechanism against emotional involvement with patients (Menzies, 1960). Although Menzies wrote this over 40 years ago, she is still widely cited by other authors when discussing the issue of nurses' emotional engagement with patients. More recently, there is evidence that nurses view emotional involvement with patients as inappropriate (Williams, 2001b). Developing partnerships with patients, however, does mean involvement. Nurses need to learn about the emotions and how to deal with them in pre-registration programmes (McQueen, 2004). Emotional labour is a neglected element of care that nurses need to learn how to deal with, and doing so will help nurses to identify and relate to patients' emotions. McQueen (2004) advocates this as the development of 'emotional intelligence'.

The emotional element in nursing is part of the 'reciprocity' component of the nurse–patient relationship or partnership, which is closely related to nursing intimacy (Muetzel, 1988). Reciprocity is where the nurse is giving of him- or herself by 'being there' for the patient. You may have been involved in situations where the patient has thanked you 'for being there'. They don't just mean that you were in the room; they felt your emotional support and were grateful for it. You did not necessarily do anything tangible. Nursing intimacy is about having close physical access and performing intimate procedures, which results in nurses being in a position to develop close emotional relationships (Williams, 2001a). Patients may tell nurses about issues they have not discussed with family or friends and, because of this, nurses are in a privileged position. This raises the question of reciprocity: how much of themselves should nurses share with patients? How can this be done in a professional and therapeutic manner? There are levels of disclosure (Williams, 2001a), which range from the exchange of superficial information ('I shop at Tesco, too') to the sharing of deeply held private secrets ('I had a miscarriage, too').

Dealing with the emotional side of nursing is demanding. As a nurse you will need to learn to cope with the stress this brings, or you may burn out and no longer be there for patients. If this happens you will not be able to help patients to participate in their care, so you need to develop strategies for de-stressing at the end of a shift and to think about how you deal with the emotional side of nursing. To help you do this, undertake Activity 3.4.

Activity 3.4   *Reflection*

- Write down what you do to reduce your stress at the end of a shift.
- What other measures do you take to cope with emotional involvement with patients?
- Look back at what you have written and decide which are positive and which are negative ways of coping with stress.
- Find out what support mechanisms are offered by your university.

An outline answer is given at the end of the chapter.

In Activity 3.4 you had the chance to think about strategies that will help you deal with the stresses that arise from engaging with patients. Writing a reflective diary may help you to explore your feelings and think about how you deal with them. You may also be able to discuss them with your tutor or mentor in supervision.

It is important not to rely on one strategy for dealing with stress, but rather to incorporate a range of them into your life. One function of the nursing handover between shifts is giving emotional support (Kerr, 2002). As nursing handovers have also been seen as a means of promoting patient participation, we will now look at how this might happen.

Handover

It is a time-honoured tradition that staff on the incoming shift must receive a report of patients' status before starting to care for them (Scovell, 2010). It is seen as time-honoured because, despite efforts to change this practice, it remains much as it has always been in some areas. Nurses also take the opportunity for some social time to catch up with their colleagues. However, we need to consider the function of handover, and how it relates to patient participation. First, it would be useful to think about your experiences and use them to analyse what the benefits and disadvantages may be of various practices.

Activity 3.5   *Communication*

1. What types of handover have you seen in practice?
2. Who was involved in these handovers?
3. Where did the handover take place?
4. Which did you think was the best, and why?

An outline answer is given at the end of the chapter.

Activity 3.5 may have helped you realise that no one method of handover is ideal. Handovers at the bedside, rather than in the office, are an opportunity to engage the patient in their care. However, patients can only be involved if they are treated as equals and the nurses fully engage with the patient. Standing at the bottom of the bed with the charts and talking from that distance will not enable the patient to offer their perspective. You may remember Hall's proxemics from psychology. The distance from the end of the bed to the patient approximates to Hall's (1966) 'social distance', that is, beyond four feet; therefore, the ensuing conversation will also be social, which will not enable patient participation. Confidentiality is also an issue: screens do not offer auditory protection, and this also may limit the discussion. The patient may feel inhibited from joining in if several nurses are involved. You may appreciate that a group of nurses talking at the bottom of the bed is not very different from the medical ward round. Indeed, Cahill talks about *maintaining professional dominance* and found that patients were very aware of the *divide between themselves and nursing staff* (1998b, p351).

Some patients did not want to be involved when they felt too ill and appreciated nurses taking over for them, but others felt that they were excluded by the use of medical jargon. You need to be very careful with the use of medical language. Imagine how upset a woman would be if she heard her diagnosis of 'spontaneous abortion' if she had just lost a much-wanted baby. While some patients found the use of language reassuring, others thought it *intolerable, dehumanizing, manipulative and controlling* (Cahill, 1998b, p355), so you need to think carefully about your use of language and how you relate to patients during handover.

Nurses do not accurately report patients' feelings, according to Cahill (1998b). Try using Hall's (1966) 'personal distance' and check out your perception of the issues with the patient. You may see them as anxious, but they may just need information about what is happening to them. You should always try to find out why a patient behaves in a challenging way. The result of not doing so is illustrated in the following case study.

Case study

Mrs Hunt, 80 years old, had been admitted for treatment of a leg ulcer. She had had diabetes for 30 years but staff thought that she must have poor understanding of the dietary requirements of her condition. In handover, it was noted that her locker was full of biscuits and sweet drinks. Each shift, the nurses commented on the fact that she had not eaten much of the food provided for her and that there were concerns about her blood sugars. After one such report, a student nurse decided to chat to Mrs Hunt and ask her why she was eating biscuits. She sat down next to her, commenced a general conversation about her hospital stay and then steered it round to the subject of food and what she was eating. Mrs Hunt explained that, because her mouth was sore, she could not manage to chew the food provided, but she knew that she must eat something and so ate the biscuits, which were soft. The student nurse asked to examine her mouth and found that it was indeed very sore and in need of care.

Labelling

The last case study demonstrates the importance of not judging or labelling patients, which may happen in handover. Patients who do not conform are often labelled as 'difficult' or 'problem patients' (Dewar and Morse, 1995). Once such labels are known, they are difficult to forget and patient care suffers. Therefore, make sure that in handover you do not make subjective or judgemental comments, and challenge any you hear. Check with the patient that assumptions made by the staff are correct. Bedside handovers are a good opportunity to do this.

Another interesting finding by Cahill (1998b) was that patients were often fed up with hearing the same details about themselves every shift change, and thought that more use could be made of documentation. In fact, they were worried that nurses didn't use the available documentation and could forget important things. Patients and nurses had different ideas about the amount of time involved in bedside handovers: nurses may think they are too time-consuming, but patients said the maximum time spent was two minutes. The study mentions that there was a good opportunity for teaching during handover, but also that this could worry patients if students lacked knowledge. Thus, it would seem that handover offers a great opportunity to promote patient participation, but that much depends on nurses' interpersonal skills.

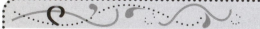

Chapter summary

This chapter has explored the meaning of patient participation and partnership, including the factors that influence it – concerning both the nurse and the patient. We have seen how nursing intimacy is beneficial for promoting participation, and how you need to consider the development of emotional intelligence, including finding ways of coping with stress.

continued opposite . . .

continued . . . •••

Respecting individuality and assessing each patient is essential, in order to determine whether they wish to participate or would prefer a more passive role. The same is true for carers and, while this has been addressed in part in this chapter, their involvement will be explored further in Chapter 4. The assessment of individual preference for participation will be explored in Chapter 6.

Activities: brief outline answers

Activity 3.1 Passive or active? (page 45)

The advantages of patients actively participating in healthcare include:

- better understanding of care;
- a sense of ownership/involvement;
- preservation of dignity;
- increased satisfaction;
- feeling that you are being respected as an individual;
- improved health education and patient adherence.

The disadvantages, i.e. patients' reasons for not wanting to participate, include:

- feeling too ill or not being bothered;
- preferring to be passive and not wanting to make decisions;
- wanting an expert to tell you what to do;
- not wanting to take responsibility for health actions;
- possibly feeling that you do not know enough and want an expert opinion;
- not being able to blame others for the outcomes of your decisions.

Activity 3.2 Partnerships (page 51)

- Types of partnership include working, business, professional, legal, sporting, social, sexual, financial and commercial.
- Attributes for a good partnership include trust, honesty, communication, respect, ability to know what the other is thinking and is wanting, negotiating skills, dependability/reliability, shared vision and goals, power sharing and equality.
- Negotiation and communication skills are central to good team working. Think what negotiation skills are. If you are negotiating your shift patterns, it means that you discuss with your mentor what would be appropriate for your learning needs and what she or he is able to supervise. You may wish to negotiate about a personal situation, but this means explaining and discussing, not telling your mentor that you cannot work a particular shift. At the end of a shift, reflect on which members of the multi-disciplinary team you have engaged with and think what went well about your communication. Make a note of key communication points that you can develop in your team working.

Activity 3.3 Multi-disciplinary meeting (page 51)

- Feelings: anxious; worried you will not understand what is said; unsure of what to expect; threatened by knowing that there will be more of them; hoping that some help may be forthcoming.
- Preparation: an agenda; need to be organised; information about different possible outcomes; knowledge of the different health and social worker roles.

Activity 3.4 Coping with stress (page 54)

• Positive strategies: listening to music, throwing bottles in a bottle bank, talking it over with family and friends, taking a walk, playing sport, having a bath, writing a diary.
• Negative strategies: drinking too much alcohol or eating excessively, driving fast, taking substances that are not healthy. You may also have thought about strategies used in practice to side-step emotional situations, such as avoiding interaction with patients.

Activity 3.5 Handover (page 55)

1. Types of handover include verbal handover, tape recordings, written handover with pre-prepared sheet, computer-generated handover.
2. Those involved could be the nurse-in-charge, a nurse looking after the group of patients, or a key worker.
3. Locations could include the patient's home, a ward or unit office, or the patient's bedside.
4. The advantages and disadvantages of the different types could include:
   – verbal handover – social and emotional contact; can ask questions but information may be lost or subjective; there may be interruptions;
   – computer-generated and tape-recorded handover – shorter and not likely to be interrupted; can be audited; no interaction, however;
   – written handover – saves time; is cost effective; again, though, no interaction.

Further reading

Bond, M (1994) *Stress and Self Awareness: A guide for nurses*. Oxford: Butterworth-Heinemann.

This book is designed to help with the stress associated with nursing and gives exercises and suggestions to enable you to develop coping strategies.

Ghaye, T and Lillyman, S (2000) *Reflection: Principles and practice for healthcare professionals*. Salisbury: Mark Allen.

This will help you to use reflection to support your insights and learning, and to develop a reflective diary as a tool for discussion with supervisors.

McQueen, A (2004) Emotional intelligence in nursing work. *Journal of Advanced Nursing*, 47: 101–8.

This is a useful review of emotional labour and intelligence, discussing their importance in nursing.

Useful websites

www.nmc-uk.org

If you access the document, *Record Keeping: Guidance for nurses and midwives* (click on 'Publications', then 'Guidance'), this will offer you direction in communicating in patient care.

www.patientopinion.org.uk

This website allows people to voice their opinions about local NHS services.

www.pickerinstitute.org.uk

The focus of this website is patient-centred care and it explores many issues surrounding this.

Chapter 4
Nursing in partnership with carers

NMC Standards for Pre-registration Nursing Education

This chapter will address the following competencies:

Domain 1: Professional values

2. All nurses must practise in a holistic, non-judgmental, caring and sensitive manner that supports social inclusion, recognises and respects individual choice and acknowledges diversity. Where necessary, they must challenge inequality, discrimination or exclusion from access to care.

4. All nurses must work in partnership with service users, carers, families, groups, communities and organisations. They must manage risk, and promote health and wellbeing while aiming to empower choices that promote self-care and safety.

5. All nurses must fully understand the nurse's various roles, responsibilities and functions, and adapt their practice to meet the changing needs of people, groups, communities and populations.

Domain 2: Communication and interpersonal skills

1. All nurses must build partnerships and therapeutic relationships through safe, effective and non-discriminatory communication. They must take account of individual differences, capabilities and needs.

4. All nurses must recognise when people are anxious or in distress and respond effectively, using therapeutic principles, to promote their wellbeing, manage personal safety and resolve conflict. They must use effective communication strategies and negotiation techniques to achieve best outcomes, respecting the dignity and human rights of all concerned. They must know when to consult a third party and how to make referrals for advocacy, mediation or arbitration.

8. All nurses must respect individual rights to confidentiality and keep information secure and confidential in accordance with the law and relevant ethical and regulatory frameworks, taking account of local protocols. They must also actively share personal information with others when the interests of safety and protection override the need for confidentiality.

NMC Essential Skills Clusters

This chapter will address the following ESCs:

Cluster: Care, compassion and communication

1. As partners in the care process, people can trust the newly registered graduate nurse to provide collaborative care based on the highest standards, knowledge and competence.

By the second progression point:

6. Forms appropriate and constructive professional relationships with families and other carers.

2. People can trust the newly registered graduate nurse to engage in person centred care, empowering people to make choices about how their needs are met when they are unable to meet them for themselves.

By the second progression point:

5. Considers with the person and their carers their capability for self-care.

By entry to the register:

13. Works autonomously, confidently and in partnership with people, their families and carers to ensure that needs are met through care planning and delivery, including strategies for self-care and peer support.

4. People can trust a newly qualified graduate nurse to engage with them and their family or carers within their cultural environments in an acceptant and anti-discriminatory manner free from harassment and exploitation.

By entry to the register:

4. Upholds people's legal rights and speaks out when these are at risk of being compromised.

7. People can trust the newly registered graduate nurse to protect and keep as confidential all information relating to them.

By the first progression point:

1. Applies the principles of confidentiality.
3. Applies the principles of data protection.

By the second progression point:

4. Distinguishes between information that is relevant to care planning and information that is not.

By entry to the register:

9. Acts within the law when confidential information has to be shared with others.

continued opposite . . .

continued . . . ●●●

Cluster: Organisational aspects of care

13. People can trust the newly registered, graduate nurse to promote continuity when their care is to be transferred to another service or person.

By the second progression point:

1. Assists people in preparing people and carers for transfer and transition through effective dialogue and giving accurate information.

Chapter aims

By the end of this chapter, you should be able to:

- define the term 'carer' and the demography of carers in the UK;
- differentiate between lay and professional caring;
- appreciate the impact of being a carer on the carer's own health;
- discuss how the nurse may promote carer partnership in nursing;
- identify sources of support for carers

Introduction

Having discussed promoting partnerships with patients in Chapter 3, we are now going to think about this in relation to their carers. First, we will look at the term 'carer' and how the term is used. Then we will analyse issues that arise from being a carer, including the impact this has on the individual socially, financially, physically and emotionally. The chapter goes on to see how the nurse and the carer should work together in caring, and what the carer wants from nurses when the patient is admitted to a healthcare setting. Finally, we will look at sources of support for carers.

Who is a carer?

First, it is important that you understand who is a carer, because this term could be confused with people employed to help people with their care. Carers in this context are not paid, but look after other people and are usually family members. Caregiving can be defined as *looking after, giving special help or some regular service that is not provided in the course of paid employment* (Hirst, 2005, p698). The carers' organisation, Carers UK, states that *Carers provide unpaid care by looking after an ill, frail or disabled family member, friend or partner* (2009, p1). As this is an unpaid activity that takes place at home, many carers do not think of themselves as being carers; they are 'just' a wife or husband or mother doing what they do. This means that figures for the number of carers are estimates.

Second, many carers do not seek help because they do not realise that being a carer entitles them to do so. They may also believe that this is their natural duty, which is called 'kinship obligation' (Deacon et al., 2008). Society expects relatives to look after each other, and older carers often feel obliged to care (Pickard et al., 2003). However, they save the NHS about £87 billion annually (Carers UK, 2010), which means that the NHS cannot afford to ignore their contribution. Let's think a little more about the characteristics of carers in Activity 4.1.

Activity 4.1   *Decision-making*

Are the following statements true or false?

1. Ten per cent of the total population are carers.   True/false
2. There are more female than male carers.   True/false
3. British men and women are more likely to be carers than their Pakistani and Bangladeshi counterparts.   True/false
4. The peak age for caring is 50 to 59.   True/false

Answers are given at the end of the chapter.

It is important to know these facts so that you are more aware of the likelihood of people being carers when you are in practice. One in eight adults is involved in caring (Carers UK, 2009), showing you that it is a common role and that you will meet many carers in nursing. There is a wide variation in the number of hours people engage in caring activity. The 2001 Census (ONS, 2001) found that six million adults over the age of 16 care for someone for more than 20 hours per week. One and a half million of these carers are looking after someone with a mental health problem (Arksey, 2003). You must also remember that children can be carers too, and we discuss their role next.

Young carers

Carers UK (2009) estimates that there are 170,000 children (under-18s) engaged in caring, usually looking after a parent or sibling. Some of these carers can be as young as four years old. In a study of what this caring involved, Lackey and Gates (2001) found that giving personal care (e.g. helping with washing and bathing) was the most frequently reported activity. Young carers also undertook household activities, medical care and social activities. Giving personal care was seen as the most difficult. Often young carers undertake these activities before and after school, which means they have a long day and very little time to themselves, which affects their school and social lives. Young carers are vulnerable to problems with their physical health, school achievement and life chances (Frank and McLarnon, 2008). They may become isolated because they lack time for leisure activities, feel that they are different from other children and have difficulty being part of a group (DH, 1999a). Young carers may not report their situation to school staff because they see school as a break from their caring (Lackey and Gates, 2001) or worry that this might result in family break-up. Therefore, school nurses should look out for children in this role.

The same study also looked at the long-term effects on young carers, and found that most of them, as adults, would let their children engage in this role, provided that they were not the sole carer (Lackey and Gates, 2001). These people had both positive and negative memories of their caring activities; further research is needed in this area.

In recognising the importance of cross-agency work to support young carers, the Department of Health (1999a) recommended that schools should designate a person to act as a link for young carers with social services, the health service and any young carers' projects. Although young carer centres are now catering for 25,000 young carers (DH, 2008b), this still leaves many unsupported.

Activity 4.2 is designed to start you thinking about the realities of caring.

Activity 4.2   *Critical thinking*

- What factors in society are increasing the number of carers?
- What would be the difference if you were caring as a lay person rather than as a nurse?

An outline answer is given at the end of the chapter.

Increased number of carers

In Activity 4.2 you might have identified the impact of changes in care provision. The increase in community care has meant that families and friends are now more involved in caregiving. Family members are now caring for people who would previously have been cared for in an institution (Wilkinson and McAndrew, 2008). Hospital stays are as short as possible, so the caring done by family members is pivotal; they are the ones who will continue to meet a patient's care needs after discharge. Collaboration between nurses and carers is essential to enable carers to carry out their role (Wilkinson and McAndrew, 2008). In children's nursing and learning disability, a family-centred approach (see Chapter 5) is widely acknowledged, but in mental health and adult nursing, it is not always adopted.

Age and relationship factors

Another factor driving up the number of carers is the ageing population; this also means that carers are often also elderly. These carers are more likely to be caring alone without other help, or having additional help available at short notice (McGarry and Arthur, 2001). It is worth remembering that there is no retirement age for caring, as Deacon et al. (2008) pointed out. Caring is more likely to be for a spouse or partner, but could be for a disabled child, or both. In a small qualitative study, McGarry and Arthur (2001) also noted that caring in later life was rarely 'unidirectional' (one-way), meaning that there was a degree of mutual support as the elderly carer may also have health needs. Together, the pair may be able to cope, but when one partner is admitted to hospital, the other may also need care because he or she cannot live unsupported. Carers often neglect their own health needs, as will be discussed later in this chapter.

You will also notice that the dependency between partners in a couple changes when one is in hospital. This 'shifting dependency' means that roles and responsibilities in the relationship also change (McGarry and Arthur, 2001). In other words, the dynamics change. This will also happen in other carer or patient relationships. A daughter may be required for the first time to carry out intimate physical care for her father, or a sister for her brother.

When you are caring for a patient, you need to consider who is caring for them when they are not in hospital. Carers' needs are often not recognised by healthcare professionals (Wollin et al., 2006).

Looking at these personal relationships shows us how the affective nature of providing care is different for family members from that of nurses. Essential professionals, such as nurses, have a functional or contractual relationship with the patient, so they are focused on directing care towards independence; the lay carer may deliver *care-giving tasks for their value as a symbol of care* (Allen, 2000, p164). When you are promoting partnership it is important that you appreciate this difference, as it is essential to be able to appreciate the view of the carer and what motivates them. In essence, they are doing it for love, while you are just doing your job. Nurses may believe in individualised care, but it is far harder to provide it in a hospital than at home. A nurse has to deal with the needs of all the patients on a ward, whereas an expert carer focuses only on their loved one (Allen, 2000). Sometimes carers express dissatisfaction when care is not of the same standard when their loved one is admitted to a hospital or nursing home. You need to understand this because, sometimes, carers will be upset and angry. Even if it seems unjustified, you need to see the situation from their perspective in order to discuss it and agree a way forward.

One other area of difference is the knowledge base. This knowledge base varies among carers according to such attributes as their level of education or financial resources, but it will also depend on the length of time they have had to build up their knowledge and how helpful healthcare professionals have been in this context. In order to appreciate the carer's needs, consider the case of Mary.

Case study

Mary was caring for her 92-year-old mother, who was becoming increasingly frail and showing signs of the onset of dementia. Her mother's increasing dependence meant that Mary had had to give up her job as a secretary to look after her mother, who, if left on her own, would turn on the gas and forget to light it. She sometimes forgot where the toilet was and, coupled with her limited mobility, this meant that she was incontinent most days. She did not sleep very much. Being confused about the time, she would call to Mary in the night to take her to the shops or start trying to make breakfast. Mary's brother lived in Australia and could not help. Mary found more and more of her time was being taken up with household activities, managing the finances and caring for her mother.

You may be able to spot some of the positive aspects of caring in this case study. Mary may feel that she is fulfilling her responsibilities as a daughter and that she can demonstrate her love for her mother by caring for her. However, it also illustrates some of the difficulties carers face. Imagine how tired Mary will be with so little sleep. As a nurse, you can go home at the end of a shift, but for Mary the shift does not end; she does not have days off. Her relationship with her brother may be adversely affected if she feels that he is not supporting her. She will have little time for herself and will probably lose friends. Social contact will become scarce, leaving Mary isolated. She has lost her job, and may have to rely on benefits, resulting in a severe loss of income. Mary will worry that, after her mother dies, she may be too old to return to work.

Effects on carer health

The above case study does not mention Mary's health, but it will doubtless be affected by undertaking this caring role. Using the General Health Questionnaire, which asks respondents about recent symptoms of psychological distress such as anxiety, Hirst (2005) found that people who undertook caring activity for 20 hours or more per week were twice as likely to show high distress scores as non-carers. These raised levels of distress were higher in women than men, and people who cared for someone in the same household, rather than in another household, were more at risk of psychological distress. In the case of carers of people with mental health problems, Ostman and Hansson (2004) supported this finding and found that distress was greater if care was given every day and if there was a longer duration of relationship. Spouse carers and mothers looking after a disabled child were most at risk of psychological distress (Hirst, 2005). These studies have found effects on the physical health of carers; half of all carers report a caring-related health condition (Cook, 2007) and all studies demonstrate risk to carers' health in the immediate period after caring ends.

Financial considerations

The caring role also affects people's finances. Many carers are unable to get or keep a job because of their caring activities. Once they cease caring, they may have difficulty, like Mary, in returning to the employment market. Carers UK (2007b) found that 72 per cent of carers suffered financially from taking on the role of carer. To appreciate the reasons for this, try Activity 4.3.

Activity 4.3   *Decision-making*

Using the internet, answer the following questions.

1. What is the carer's allowance?
2. Are there any restrictions on receiving it?
3. What other financial implications are there of being a carer?
4. Do carers claim all their financial entitlements and, if not, why not?
5. How much is it estimated that carers save the taxpayer annually?
6. How do you think you would manage on the above allowances?

Outline answers are given at the end of the chapter.

From looking at the figures, you can see why carers may have financial difficulties, which place further strain on them. Some of this financial strain arises because many carers have to alter their working patterns or give up work. Carers UK (2007a) found that 54 per cent of carers had given up work to care, many retiring early – on average by eight years. To understand the experience of caring further, consider the following life stories.

Being a carer

Activity 4.4   *Critical thinking*

Carl gave up work to look after his wife, Daphne, when they were both in their fifties. She had suffered from severe depression for a number of years, which had resulted in frequent hospitalisations. Carl's action did have the result he wanted, which was a reduction in this revolving-door experience of hospitalisation, day care and home.

Fourteen years ago, Daphne needed major bowel surgery, which resulted in a rapid transit ileostomy. Carl found that she was well looked after in hospital, with staff appearing to appreciate his role as her carer due to her severe depression. However, they did not involve him in her stoma care. So, on discharge, he was given a bag full of stoma care equipment but only 15 minutes' training in how to use it. There was a bank holiday weekend coming up and he did not feel at all confident that he would be able to manage without support.

1. How do you think Carl felt?
2. What issues did Carl identify as important?
3. What could nurses have done to help Carl in this situation?

An outline answer, supplied by Carl, is given at the end of the chapter.

Case study

Anam's earliest memory of caring is when she was eight. She recalls sitting on a wall watching over her two brothers, Yousif and Imran, who both have learning difficulties. She wanted to go and play with her friends but had been told by her parents that she must look out for her brothers.

For the last 14 years, she has become their main carer. Her brothers can vacuum, make cups of tea and get themselves dressed, but need assistance with all these activities. Anam cares for them as well as being a mother to her own children, who are aged 20, 14 and 10. At first she found caring daunting, but then realised that people all have good qualities whether they are disabled or able-bodied. What was important was to recognise this. Her children have after-school activities and are doing well, as are her brothers, who like to play snooker and ball games. She says that caring is hard and, at first, she found her brothers' behaviour difficult to handle.

continued opposite . . .

continued . . .

Then, she and some other carers set up a local action group because they were not being listened to nor getting the information they wanted. She describes the group as a 'big family' who go on outings together and support each other. Anam states that she feels now she can achieve whatever goal she sets herself. She has become involved in educational activities with nursing students and has written a chapter for a textbook. Anam says, For me, caring is empowering – caring is all about love.

Anam's story illustrates both the positive and negative sides of caring. It also shows how carers may look after more than one person and have to juggle the differing needs of family members. Sometimes referred to as the 'sandwich generation', these carers have responsibilities both to elderly parents and to children with special needs.

These scenarios are based on real lives and show the positive as well as the challenging sides of being a carer. They also demonstrate how caring is not separated into the fields of nursing and, therefore, you always need to assess care needs holistically. Where you feel unable to meet a patient's needs yourself, refer to an appropriate professional and work together to address these; interprofessional working is important here. Carers value support and need information in order to carry out their role.

In Anam's scenario, there could have been cultural issues. Female carers of some South Asian families cannot rely on help from other family members, as touching is prohibited between adult family members who are not married (Deacon et al., 2008). This study looked at gender issues and culture, finding that male carers were more likely to receive support from family members than female carers. Also, South Asian women may find obtaining help from social services more difficult because of language and communication problems. These, however, were not issues for Anam.

You need to acknowledge the needs of carers and be careful not to make assumptions, for example that a carer has no need for help because they have the support of an extended family. Be sensitive also to carers who are gay or lesbian, as they may experience difficulties when one is hospitalised. If there is no civil partnership, the other person will not be regarded as next of kin. Remember that they may have 'come out' in the wider world but be embarrassed to do so in hospital. Also, carers may not be caring for just one person – they could be multiple carers. The sandwich generation may be caring for a child with special needs as well as an elderly parent. You must assess all carers as individuals, and explore what they, not you, see as their needs.

You may wish to find out more about carers' experiences in your field of nursing and, to do this, you could undertake Activity 4.5.

Activity 4.5   *Reflection*

Access **www.patientvoices.org.uk** and look at carers' stories, or go to **www.carers uk.org**, click on 'Forums' and read some of the blogs.

continued overleaf . . .

continued . . .

Try to consider how you would feel if you were in these carers' situations. Would you suffer financially or physically and could this lead to social exclusion?

This is for individual reflection and no outline answer is provided.

Carers and health professionals

Now that we have explored some of the issues of being a carer, we can discuss what they need from healthcare professionals, and from nurses in particular. As we saw, there is a difference in the knowledge base among carers. Some may have explored and developed their knowledge base, for example by taking a moving and handling course to enable them to move a handicapped child in a manner that is safe for both of them. Others may be seeking knowledge. What carers have, however, is an intimate knowledge of the person that they are caring for. Carers want to work in partnership with nurses (Wilkinson and McAndrew, 2008), but they need nurses to value their knowledge in order for this partnership to be created. Ignoring this knowledge will be detrimental to the patient, as evidenced in the following case study.

Case study

Irene was 88 years old and lived by herself in a sheltered flat. She was suffering from COPD (chronic obstructive pulmonary disease) and becoming a little confused at times, but with the support of her daughter, who called at least twice a day and did her shopping and cooking, she managed. Her daughter helped her bathe and meet her hygiene needs, and she had a cleaner once a week. Irene suffered an episode of acute breathlessness and was admitted to a medical ward. The daughter asked her nurse if her mobility could be maintained by encouraging her to walk to the toilet, as she was concerned that her mother would lose her ability to do this while in hospital and be unable to return to her flat.

When the daughter visited her the next day, the nurse said that they had tried to mobilise her to the toilet, but she had become very breathless and her oxygen saturations had dropped to 85 per cent. Since then, they had administered oxygen, kept her by her bed and brought her the commode when required. The daughter asked where the toilet was and was told, 'Oh, just down that corridor at the end.' This made the daughter realise that her mother had been asked to walk many times further than she did in her own flat and it was no wonder she became breathless. She had not walked that far in years. No one had thought to ask how far her mother normally walked. Her mother was discharged a couple of weeks later, but her mobility and mental state had deteriorated so much that, within three months, she was admitted to a nursing home.

The above scenario shows what can happen when the nurse fails to obtain essential information about activities of living from a carer when the patient is unable to provide it. While assessment will be discussed in Chapter 6, carer perspectives on their involvement in assessments will be discussed later in this chapter.

When the person they are caring for is in a healthcare setting, carers want to work collaboratively (Wilkinson and McAndrew, 2008). They need to maintain some element of control, in order to sustain their resilience to cope with caring, and collaborating in the treatment process is an important way of doing this. All carers in a study expressed a desire for partnership. One informant said, *it's about working together, the team knowing that I have valuable things to contribute and vice versa, because we all want the same at the end of the day* (Wilkinson and McAndrew, 2008, p397). Yet informants also expressed a sense of powerlessness and isolation, with one informant saying, *As soon as he was admitted to the ward, I became a nobody, an outsider, but I am not an outsider, I am his mother* (ibid.). It may seem strange that healthcare professionals would seek to exclude a carer from the care setting when it is on the carer that the patient will depend when discharged. Carers want to contribute and have a need to be informed about treatment. Activity 4.6 is designed to enable you to focus on your approach to carer involvement.

Activity 4.6   *Communication*

You are sitting with Mr Jones, who has had a cerebro-vascular accident, helping him to eat his dinner. His wife arrives and says that he can manage to swallow better if you put the food into the right side of his mouth rather than centrally. Also, he needs to be reminded to swallow after each mouthful. How do you react?

Do you:

a. pretend you did not hear and carry on regardless;
b. say that hospital policy states that you must do it in the way you are doing;
c. invite Mrs Jones to show you what she means;
d. listen patiently and try to do what she says;
e. think that she should leave this to you and be grateful for the respite.

Descriptions of each of these strategies are provided at the end of the chapter.

Sometimes, we do not always stop to reflect on why we act the way we do or think of the consequences of our response for carers. If a situation makes you uncomfortable, you may seek to avoid it, especially when you do not feel confident in your practice or feel that you are being challenged. Nurses, despite knowing that carers are experts, find it hard to accept advice from them without feeling that their professional knowledge is compromised (Allen, 2000). While she found that carers were mostly permitted to stay during caregiving activities, Allen observed that this left nurses *feeling exposed, particularly unqualified staff who, unlike professional nurses, could not lay claim to officially sanctioned expertise* (2000, p159).

Valuing carer knowledge

Sometimes, hospital staff, especially those with less training, may feel that they are being criticised and their expertise questioned by the contribution of carers. Nurses rarely proactively seek a carer's input and, as a result of this, carers find it difficult to contribute without feeling that they are criticising (Allen, 2000). Nursing teams need to adopt a philosophy of valuing the contribution of carers, and recognising its worth. Time and again we hear that carers need to be valued and have their role respected by healthcare professionals. Carers want their knowledge of the patient recognised, and for nurses to appreciate the emotional impact caused by hospital admission (Wilkinson and McAndrew, 2008). Once carers feel that their worth is acknowledged, they feel supported (Deacon et al., 2008). In another study, carers said they wanted their contribution to be recognised because they felt that this was not always the case and, consequently, they also felt ignored during consultations (McGarry and Arthur, 2001). You need, therefore, to acknowledge the expertise of the carer and see their role as complementary rather than challenging.

Carers also need information and knowledge about treatment. Without this, carers feel a sense of powerlessness and loss of control (Wilkinson and McAndrew, 2008). Once the person they care for enters hospital, they feel a sense of 'us' and 'them' rather than partnership, with the professionals having all the knowledge and control. *Knowledge is a source of power and not sharing information with carers disempowers them, leaving health-care professionals free to maintain control over decision-making* (Wilkinson and McAndrew, 2008, p398).

Don't let information or knowledge be a source of contention. Carers sometimes feel that they are excluded on the grounds of confidentiality. While acknowledging confidentiality, carers need information to be able to care when the patient is discharged.

Confidentiality and informed consent

Confidentiality is a complex issue. By law and in your professional code of conduct, you are required to maintain patient confidentiality and can face disciplinary action for breaking it. This also applies to respecting carer confidentiality. Carers may be concerned about reporting patient symptoms to you for fear of the impact this may have on their relationship with the patient, who may see it as a breach of confidentiality. However, the Department of Health (2003a) clearly states that issues around confidentiality should not be used as a reason for not listening to carers or sharing information with them. It is important that you work with patients and carers to establish consent for information to be shared. Not all patients and carers are aware of the centrality of consent in information-sharing, so you need to discuss the issue of confidentiality at an early stage. Encourage the use of advance directives as the patient's condition, for example dementia, may deteriorate to the extent that they are not able to give consent. Advance directives allow patients, when they are fit enough to do so, to plan what they want to happen should they become unwell. Make sure that all issues concerning confidentiality are recorded in the patient's notes and are part of the care plan signed by the patient.

You should encourage patients to see the benefits of sharing information appropriately. Sometimes, patients may be reluctant to do this, in which case sit down with them and explore their reasons. It may be that there is some piece of information that is particularly sensitive and that they wish to keep private. In this case, agreement could be reached about what is and what is not shared. You could try talking to the patient on their own, then the carer on their own, and then together, to harmonise the process and ensure that all parties have the opportunity to establish what is sensitive, personal and not for sharing, as opposed to what is general and can be shared. Do not withold general information from carers on the grounds of confidentiality. Most Trusts have leaflets explaining these issues for patients and carers, so look out for these when you are in practice and read them.

Support

Case study

At a carers' centre, the following answers were given to the author's questions.

1. **What do you need from nurses when your loved one is in hospital?**
   - *Recognition of the emotions we are feeling – powerlessness, loss of control, guilt. Don't denigrate us as being over-anxious and say things like 'Relax, we know what we are doing', because carers do fret about whether care will be given in the way we would give it.*
   - *Actively listen to us so that you appreciate our needs. If a carer has been staying with a sick child, they may appreciate your offering to give them a break by sitting with their child.*
   - *We need to be involved – don't exclude us. Ask us to show you how we would do things.*
   - *When loved ones cannot communicate, we worry that you will understand when they are uncomfortable. Be flexible with visiting and allowing carers to stay.*
   - *Remember older carers may be afraid to ask – they come from a generation who did not question healthcare professionals.*
   - *Appreciate the fear that the strange environment causes. You are used to all the equipment but it is frightening to us.*
   - *We need information and complete explanations. One carer had been told that her daughter's oxygen must be delivered at 1.5 litres. She thought that if it dropped to one litre, her daughter would die.*
   - *Recognise added financial implications of hospitalisation such as parking, telephone calls, food while visiting.*
   - *Respect family relationships and do not judge carers' reactions to other family members, such as protecting some members. These family dynamics will exist after discharge.*

2. **In general, what are your biggest concerns?**
   - *Better financial help.*
   - *Short-term breaks.*
   - *Better information about and finance of long-term care.*
   - *Flexibility.*

It is interesting to compare these local views with those of a research study.

Research summary: 'How do we facilitate carers' involvement in decision-making?' (Walker and Dewar, 2001)

Aim: to explore carer involvement in a specific care context to identify opportunities for change.

Policy documents have made statements about involvement without addressing fundamental questions about how such policies should be implemented.
(p334)

Method: a qualitative case study design using audio-taped semi-structured interviews and focus groups.

Sample: 20 carers and 29 members of the multi-disciplinary team in a 23- bedded mental health unit.

Data analysis: constant comparative analysis (Glaser and Strauss, 1967).

Findings: carer dissatisfaction with their level of involvement. Two sources of difficulty for this were identified:

a. Hospital systems and processes. *Professionals were unaware of the ways in which carers were oppressed by hospital systems they took for granted* (p333). Familiarity with these enabled professionals to dominate procedures such as discharge planning.
b. Relationship between hospital staff and carers. Staff had difficulty coping with carer demands and labelled them as *guilt ridden and emotionally vulnerable.*

This led to problems in the relationship with staff seeking to avoid them rather than involve them, as staff found contact with carers stressful.

Four markers of satisfactory involvement:

1. *feeling information is shared;*
2. *feeling included in decision making;*
3. *feeling that there is someone you can contact when you need to;*
4. *feeling that the service is responsive to your needs.*
   (p332)

Conclusion: level and nature of involvement of carers varied according to the practice of individual staff members.

How can you use these findings in your practice? You need to show carers around the ward area and explain procedures to them – to orientate them, which will make the environment seem less strange. This will help them to feel more at ease. Take time to listen to them and show that you value their opinions by the use of non-verbal cues such as body language, as well as verbal communication. Reflect on your practice to make sure that you are not avoiding contact with carers and, if you find this stressful, think of the strategies discussed in the previous chapter for dealing with emotional labour. Seek permission from the patient and involve carers throughout the patient's stay, making sure that they are fully informed. Allow them time to ask questions.

Carers need emotional support, and value *having someone with whom they could talk* (Nolan and Dellasega, 2000, p764). In a study of three groups of carers – those of older people, carers of technology-dependent children and home-care workers, Pickard et al. (2003) found that the key role of nurses should be in information-giving and offering emotional support. Emotional support is particularly important when the carer is facing the loss of the person they knew, which can happen suddenly when an individual develops a health problem such as a stroke or when their mental capacity deteriorates and they no longer recognise the person caring for them. Think how distressing it must be to become a stranger to the person you have loved for a long time. Nurses need to offer this support for lay carers so that they became confident in their caregiving. Carers do want their emotional needs to be addressed by nurses and support offered (Wilkinson and McAndrew, 2008). Carers UK (2010) identified three main ways in which the NHS should help carers:

1. identify carers and proactively support them in their caring role;
2. provide training for carers;
3. treat carers as partners in providing care.

Information about national sources of information set up in line with DH strategy (2008b) can be found at the end of the chapter.

One form of support that is available to carers is a health needs assessment. Carers are legally entitled to this assessment, which is designed to identify both their requirements and those of the cared-for person (Community Care and Health Act 2002). This assessment should look at whether the carer wishes to continue in this role and, if so, establish what would help them, such as equipment or breaks. It should assess whether the carer wants to work and/or take part in leisure or education. There should be discussion of what service options there are and a plan for what would happen in an emergency. Employment law does differ across the UK. Carers may not know of their right to a health assessment but, equally, an assessment will only help if the identified needs are then met. Further information on health assessment and how you can help carers to access them can be found on the websites given at the end of the chapter.

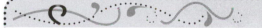

Chapter summary

As a nurse, you have a responsibility to identify carers as they often do not think of themselves in this way. Patient assessment, which will be discussed in Chapter 6, offers an opportunity for this and for you to focus on the whole family (see Chapter 5). You need to work with carers as partners in care who support each other and respect each other's knowledge, valuing their contribution. In Chapter 1, you were encouraged to think *Who is this person and how must they be feeling?* (Johns, 1991, p1095), but you should also consider who is their carer and how they must be feeling. The government vision for 2018 (DH, 2008b) for carers to become expert care partners will only become reality if every nurse works to achieve this partnership.

Activities: brief outline answers

Activity 4.1 Carer statistics (page 62)

1. True: in England and Scotland, 10 per cent of the total population are carers; in Northern Ireland and Wales, this is 11 per cent.
2. True: the 2001 Census shows that 58 per cent of carers are female.
3. False: Bangladeshi and Pakistani men and women are three times more likely to be carers than their British counterparts.
4. True: this is the peak age for carers, with one and a half million in this age group.

(Source: Carers UK, 2010.)

Activity 4.2 The realities of caring (page 63)

*   The NHS Information Centre estimates that the number of people caring for more than 50 hours has doubled in nine years. The ageing population is increasing. Advances in medicine mean more people are surviving with disabilities. Government policy means that more people in all fields of nursing are being cared for in the community while hospital provision is reduced.
*   **Lay carers** – emotional involvement with patient, personal relationship, two-way relationship, knowledge, time commitment, financial issues.
    Professionals – different knowledge base, contact during shifts, professional relationship from nurse to patient.

Activity 4.3 Financial considerations (page 65)

1. The carer's allowance is currently £53.09p. Claiming the carer's allowance may entitle you to other state benefits. Benefits may vary between England, Wales, Scotland and Northern Ireland.
2. You must be 16 years or over; you must care for 35 hours minimum per week; the person you look after must receive a qualifying disability benefit; you cannot earn more than £100 per week; you must not be a full-time student; and you must not be claiming certain other benefits, e.g. state pension.
3. Respite care, special equipment, diet, for example.
4. No. Many are unaware of potential benefits or find it too difficult to claim. Carers UK estimates that there is £740 million of unclaimed benefit. Further information on finance can be found at **www.carersuk.org**.
5. It is currently estimated that carers save the taxpayer £87 billion a year.

Activity 4.4 Carl's experience as carer (page 66)

1. Carl said he felt anxious, daunted, frustrated and unsupported.
2. Lack of information on what will happen after discharge, such as how to get help out of hours. Lack of proper initial training and ongoing support in the use of equipment.
3. They could have included him with Daphne in learning about stoma care and how to deal with the stress of the situation, and could have offered ongoing sources of support.

Activity 4.6 Mr and Mrs Jones (page 69)

The five choices (a–e) can be described as follows.

a. Carers report feeling excluded (Wilkinson and McAndrew, 2008).
b. This would be seen as exerting control (Allen, 2000).
c. This would be seen as encouraging participation.
d. This would be seen as being supportive.
e. This assumes that you know what the carer wants, but the carer may feel guilty about not caring for her husband or may feel that she still wants to do as much as she can for him.

Further reading

Department of Health (DH) (1999) *National Strategy for Carers.* London: Department of Health. Available online at **www.dh.gov.uk**.

This contains practice recommendations for healthcare professionals concerning both adult and young carers. See appendix one for helplines for carers and appendix three for other support services.

Department of Health (DH) (2003) *Confidentiality: NHS code of practice.* London: Department of Health.

This contains further guidance on patient and carer confidentiality.

Department of Health (DH) (2008) *Carers at the Heart of 21st-century Families and Communities.* London: Department of Health. Available online at **www.dh.gov.uk**.

This is the government's short-term agenda and long-term vision for the future care and support of carers.

Jordan, M (2006) *The Essential Carer's Guide.* London: Princess Royal Trust for Carers.

This contains chapters with information on various subjects that carers need, such as skin care.

Monroe, B and Oliviere, D (2003) *Patient Participation in Palliative Care: A voice for the voiceless.* Oxford: Oxford University Press.

This book will help you to think about carers' needs when they lose the person they are caring for.

Useful websites

www.carers.org

This is the Princess Royal Trust for Carers, which supplies information, advice and support services through a network of over 100 independently managed carers' centres across the UK.

www.carersuk.org

This website is designed and maintained by Carers UK, which is an organisation set up to champion carers and to give the voiceless a voice. It seeks to influence policy and promote carers' rights. You can read carers' stories here. There are separate websites for Scotland, **www.carersscotland.org**, Wales, **www.carers wales.org**, and Northern Ireland, **www.carersni.org**. On this site, you can find carer health assessment information, including a sample letter of application.

www.crossroads.org.uk

Also available in Northern Ireland, **www.crossroadcare.co.uk**, and Scotland, **www.crossroads-scotland.co.uk**, these schemes provide a range of services for carers, including within the home to enable carers to have a break.

www.dh.gov.uk

Look under the 'Carers' information section (found under 'Social care') for all the support and rights of carers. Also, access NHS Choices.

www.nhsdirect.nhs.uk

This site provides helplines for carers and covers a range of different conditions.

www.rcpsych.ac.uk

This contains further information on carers and confidentiality in mental health.

www.youngcarer.com

This is a useful site for young carers covering a range of subjects and containing young carer blogs.

www.youngcarers.net

This is an online service for young carers from the Princess Royal Trust, which allows young people to search for young carers' projects and support groups by postcode.

Chapter 5
Family-centred care

Melanie Robbins

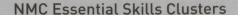

NMC Essential Skills Clusters

This chapter will address the following ESCs:

Cluster: Organisational aspects of care

9. People can trust the newly registered graduate nurse to treat them as partners and work with them to make a holistic and systematic assessment of their needs; to develop a personalised plan that is based on mutual understanding and respect for their individual situation, promoting health and well-being, minimising risk of harm and promoting their safety at all times.

By the second progression point:

10. With the person and under supervision, plans safe and effective care by recording and sharing information based on the assessment.

12. In partnership with the person, their carers and their families, makes a holistic, person centred and systematic assessment of physical, emotional, psychological, social, cultural and spiritual needs, including risk, and together, develops a comprehensive personalised plan of nursing care.

11. People can trust the newly registered graduate nurse to safeguard children and adults from vulnerable situations and support and protect them from harm.

By the second progression point:

4. Documents concerns and information about people who are in vulnerable situations.

By entry to the register:

5. Recognises and responds when people are in vulnerable situations and at risk, or in need of support and protection.

6. Shares information safely with colleagues and across agency boundaries for the protection of individuals and the public.

Chapter aims

By the end of this chapter, you should be able to:

- understand the importance of attachment;
- define family-centred care;
- outline the responsibilities of all nursees when working with children and families;
- appreciate the importance of partnership in safeguarding situations, when professionals have additional responsibility.

Introduction

In this chapter we will explore what is meant by family and family-centred care (FCC). Many health and social care workers state that they do not look after children, but leave care to those with special training, such as children's nurses, social workers and teachers. This view is outdated. Whenever you work with an adult who has a family with children, what you do will affect a child, so you are working *with* children. This goes for other dependent relatives as well. When considering the care needs of an adult, you need to consider how their role as mother, father, grandparent, aunt/uncle or carer affects their ability to continue to support the needs of the children or other dependants in that household.

Such dependants may have additional care needs: they may have disabilities, life-limiting illnesses or complex health needs, for example. The Children Act 1989 clearly states that the child's needs are paramount and the Children Act 2004 states that every professional has a legal duty to report any concerns they have about a child's welfare. Meeting the care needs of children is the responsibility of all health and social care workers; even if your role may only be to refer the child and family to other services that can support them, you must include the child's needs in any assessment. FCC also takes into consideration the needs of other family members, including elderly relatives.

Attachment

When working with children it is important to consider the whole family. Children do not live in isolation and, depending on their age and cognitive and physical abilities, may rely on their family to provide for their needs and to make decisions for them. Early work by researchers highlighted the negative impact on a child's development, both physically and emotionally, that family separation such as an admission to hospital can have. Bowlby's work (1969, 1973, 1980) showed that children need an 'attachment figure' to provide emotional security when they feel threatened or anxious. More recent work demonstrates that a child needs to develop a limited number of 'strong attachments' with those who provide care, to enable the child to grow emotionally. These people can be of either gender. Coupled with a stimulating environment, the way the attachment figure responds to the child's needs provides the emotional and physical security children need to feel confident to explore their environment, fostering their cognitive and physical development. The recognition that this attachment is important for development has underpinned research studies addressing the impact of alternative childcare on very young children. For each study that states that young children are not adversely affected by such provision, another suggests that very young children *are* affected (Ahnert et al., 2006).

What is 'family'?

Activity 5.1   *Reflection*

What do we mean when we talk about the family? How would you define a family?

This is for individual reflection and no outline answer is provided.

As you will have considered in Activity 5.1, families are very diverse and do not all follow the stereotype of mum, dad, two children and the golden labrador, as commonly portrayed in the media. Families do not function in isolation and there are many influences that need to be considered when trying to understand how a family works, such as history and values passed on between generations, and the influences of society and cultural norms, which may support the continuation of values, but may also challenge and modify values between generations. Hemphill and Dearmum (2006) suggest that it is the family that defines itself and a more pertinent question for nurses to ask is, who is part of any particular family?

Activity 5.2   *Reflection*

Who is in your family and who offers you support?

1. First, draw a circle and write your name in it to represent you. Name all the people you consider as family and put them outside and around the circle, and link each individual to you by a connecting line. Are all the people related to you, or are there names of people who are unrelated to you?
2. Now, consider who you receive support from; if the person provides you with a lot of support make the line wider; for those people who only offer you a little support, keep the line a thin one. You may have identified people who offer support in different areas of your life, e.g. your tutor from your course, your pastor or priest, your next-door neighbour or your friend from school. Look at your diagram; where do you draw your support from, are they all relatives or are there friends in there as well?
3. You can also indicate the flow of support on the line by placing a directional arrow, indicating you receiving or giving support. Why do you think it is important to understand where people gain their support?

An outline answer is given at the end of the chapter.

The type of diagram you have drawn in Activity 5.2 is called an ecomap and it enables you to find out who is giving support to a family, and who the family is supporting, so that care can be planned to maintain or support these links. An ecomap enables you to view who is in the family system, and explore the interactions and relationships within it by following the flow of support – important information for planning care (Rempel et al., 2007).

Wright and Leahey (1994) suggest viewing families as systems that work together. When one part of the system is altered, such as by illness, the system is changed and interaction between members of the system will be affected. Healthcare professionals work towards rebalancing the system by addressing the imbalance or helping the system to reconfigure. The diagram in Activity 5.3 shows an ecomap, which enables you to view who is in the family system, and to explore the interactions and relationships within that family by following the flow of support – important information for planning care (Rempel et al., 2007).

Activity 5.3   *Decision-making*

What do you think you need to consider when planning care for the family in the following ecomap?

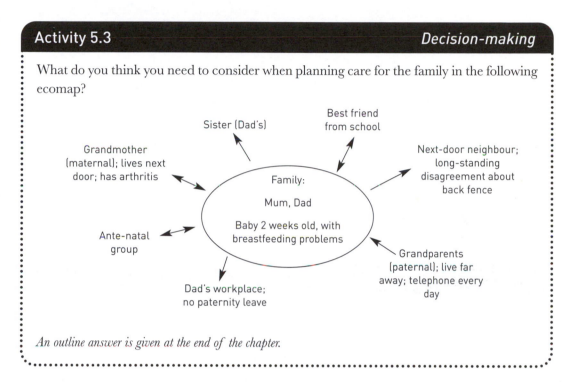

An outline answer is given at the end of the chapter.

Understanding who supports a person and how, and who is the most important person to them, are vital when you develop a care plan that draws on those support networks appropriately. You have explored some of these issues in previous chapters. As nurses, we cannot assume we know who are the most important people in a patient's support network, nor ignore our patients' responsibilities to others in that network.

Attachment and separation in a health context

Robertson and Robertson's work (1955, 1970, and a series of films, 1967–71) identified children's responses to separation from their attachments, starting with protest and then progressing through the stages to the end stage, where the child is unable to interact with the mother and rejects any attempt to re-establish a relationship. The stages are:

- protest (but child is able to be comforted);
- despair (child is inconsolable);
- denial/detachment (child appears to be unconcerned about the separation, then appears to reject the mother on reunion).

The series of five films showing the separation process (*Young Children in Brief Separation*) is very powerful. The story of John shows a young boy who is cared for in an LA care home, while this mother has a second child. John clearly demonstrates separation protest and his anguish is still fresh in my mind, some 28 years after I first viewed the film. The effects of that experience continued to show in his behaviour for a considerable time. However, studies found that regular visits or stays by the child's mother or other attachment figure, including the father, helped to reduce a child's distress.

Family-centred care

The way we work with families in both healthcare and social work has completely changed since the beginning of 1900s, when a child would be left alone in hospital with brief visits from their parents. Following the Second World War, interest in the effects of separation meant that an ever-increasing number of children's hospitals began to allow parents to visit daily. Nowadays it is normal for a parent to stay with the child, and this change was greatly influenced by the work of the Robertsons, which showed that a child who has a parent with them is better able to cope with any anxiety or even pain. This 'family-centred care (FCC)' developed from an understanding of the importance of providing a 'consistent carer' to ensure a child's continued well-being.

Activity 5.4　　　　　　　　　　　　　　　　　　*Reflection*

Try to imagine yourself as a young child going into hospital for the first time (you may have actually experienced this in your childhood). How do you think you would feel?

This is for individual reflection, but read on for further discussion.

You may have imagined feelings of anxiety, your senses assaulted by new sounds, new smells and lots of new people. This may be in addition to feeling pain because of the reason you are in hospital in the first place. You may have already had experiences of hospital before that inform your perspective now.

As the professional looking after a young child, what do you think you would want to know, and what would you need to have?

Research tells us that patients want information that is accurate and given in a timely manner (Caress, 2003). Children are no different in this, but they need information they can understand. Nurses have to be careful, though, with certain phrases: we may talk about a child having a 'special sleep' to explain an anaesthetic, but a child may have heard that pets also have a 'special sleep' at the vet's and know they do not come back.

Case study

Ben, aged five, needs to come into hospital for routine dental extraction. His experience of hospitals started 18 months ago when he came to visit his Gran, who died two days later. Six months later, he visited his uncle, who had been in a road traffic incident but was recovering well, but then acquired MRSA and died from an overwhelming infection. Both Ben's parents view the hospital with suspicion and a little dread.

Activity 5.5 — *Communication*

- How do you think Ben in the last case study is feeling about his 'routine' procedure?
- What would you want to help you cope with this experience?
- As Ben's nurse, how would you approach the family?

An outline answer is given at the end of the chapter.

Communication skills are vital here. Ben needs to be reassured that a hospital visit does not always end in death. He may also need the opportunity to explore any feelings of loss he may have but not be able to label; this is an important process, and play or art therapy can be useful here. His mum and dad may also need help and support to enable Ben to talk about his fears, as concepts of death and loss can also be difficult for adults. They may also have their own fears about Ben's routine procedure, given the family's experiences of healthcare so far. Keeping Ben's routines as normal as possible will help to reduce the number of 'new' experiences Ben has to process, and will provide him with familiarity and comfort. Knowing that at least one of his parents will be with him throughout the stay enables Ben to receive reassurance and love whenever he needs it.

Having a parent there to help reassure and maintain the things that are normal helps to reduce a child's anxiety level. Normal activities, such as the child's bedtime routine, and getting up, washed and dressed in the morning, are important as these reduce the newness of the experience and are the easiest ways of including the family in a child's care.

We do not always recognise the importance of familiarity when working with adults. In an adult hospital ward, it may not be easy for a member of the family to stay with an adult patient, even if they have been that person's main and constant carer for a number of years. Changes in routine are frightening and confusing for some adult patients too.

Scenario

Imagine you, as a student nurse, are on practice learning experience in an adult ward. The staff are open to any new ideas you may have. What simple changes could you suggest that may make the adult environment more accessible for carers to stay for longer?

Degree of involvement

FCC is part of the discussion about the degree of family involvement in care. Is such involvement a participation or a partnership? And to what extent is the partnership led by the patient or carer? You may like to look back at the concepts of participation and partnership in Chapter 3.

Case study

Janet has one child at home, aged 18 months, and she has given birth to a little boy, Sean, seven weeks prematurely. Sean is being nursed in the SCBU in an incubator, as he has had some difficulty breathing and is receiving oxygen via a nasal probe. He is fed two-hourly via a nasogastric tube to reduce his oxygen demands and prevent him becoming too tired. Janet cannot live in with Sean because of her other child at home, so most of his care needs are delivered by the nurses. Janet feels that the nurses expect her to get involved with Sean's care, but with all the tubes and alarms she is frightened she may do something wrong. Also, most of Sean's care needs (washing, nappy changing) are done by the nurses by the time she arrives at the unit.

Activity 5.6   *Critical thinking*

- How do you think Janet feels about her role as a mum?
- What do you think the nurses feel about Janet?
- What would you suggest to help the situation?

An outline answer is given at the end of the chapter.

We can be guilty of assuming that, because families attend to their child's day-to-day needs at home, they are willing and able to do so in hospital. We are very used to working with children and babies who have lots of technical equipment to aid their care and may fail to see how frightening this may be for parents. Care for children with more complex needs has also developed significantly over the last decade. More children with conditions that would have been fatal in earlier years are now living longer with greater technological support (Hewitt-Taylor, 2005). This care can be delivered in hospital, but many aspects of care are now delivered in the child's home, for example ventilation support, or complex medication regimes delivered by central lines. While there is nursing support, the majority of care for these children is delivered by families. Parents may feel pressured to learn skills previously considered nursing skills, but what is their role here – as a parent or as a nurse?

In busy ward environments, it is easy for nurses to view parents as part of the workforce because, if parents were not there, nurses would be very hard pressed to be able to deliver care for the whole ward. Conversely, for some students in children's nursing, it is quite a shock to find that they won't be caring for the infants; rather, that their role is to help parents give that care. Key here is your role in assessing the child and family to ensure that the level of involvement is right for them; ask them to do too much and you may be adding to the pressure on the family system, with parents feeling pressured, frightened and anxious about some of the tasks they feel you want them to do. Alternatively, not involving them in their child's care may also create pressure in the family system, as parents may feel sidelined and excluded.

There are similarities when working with adults and their carers; the latter may feel pressurised into engaging in care because of family ties and a sense of duty. Once patients are admitted to hospital, we need to ensure that carers are as involved in the delivery of care as they wish to be.

Case study

Alan, aged 13, has complex healthcare needs and struggles to eat, as his swallowing reflex is affected by neurological problems. He arrives on the ward and, following assessment, it is clear that he is losing weight. He has been staying with his dad for the weekend; his parents are divorced but have joint parental responsibility. The doctors suggest that Alan has a gastrostomy tube fitted to help him supplement his nutritional intake. His dad agrees that this would be a good idea; however, when his mum arrives she says she doesn't want Alan to have a gastrostomy because, when she has him, she makes sure he eats enough, even if it takes over an hour for him to feed. She implies that dad doesn't have the patience to sit with Alan and help him to feed.

Activity 5.7   *Critical thinking*

Who are we in partnership with in the case study above, in the case of Alan and his parents?

This is for individual reflection, but read on for further discussion.

In this situation we are in fact working with both parents, and the role of the nurse is to consider both of their needs in the context of meeting Alan's needs. Both may have very valid reasons for their decision about the best way to care for Alan. Parents do not have to be separated or divorced to have differing views on care choices. This is also true of carers for adults. Siblings may not agree the course of treatment for their elderly father; one may wish to look after him at home, while the other may prefer him to go into a nursing home.

We do not have a crystal ball to look back into a family's history, and how relationships have grown or have been challenging. Hurts and affirmations can challenge or support relationships and these influence a carer's choices, either consciously or not. The person being cared for may also have clear views, which are important. In the case study, the person we have not heard from is Alan.

At 13 years, Alan is old enough to understand some of the implications of care decisions and he may have his own very clear view as to whether to have a gastrostomy or not. A nurse working with children needs to understand the level of cognitive development the child has reached and whether it is appropriate to involve them in their care decisions. This right is set out within the

United Nations Convention on the Rights of the Child (UNCRC) of 1989, the Children Act 1989 and in many policy documents relating to the care of children. Be aware that parents may struggle to accept that their 'child' can make the right decisions for themselves. In this situation you have to work with care and consideration for all involved.

Participation and partnership

The difference between participation and partnership is to do with who is perceived to have the power in a relationship. A patient who has participation in care still has care that is nurse-led; ideally, in the case of a child, the parents decide how much they become involved in care delivery, but the decision may still lie with the nurse. In partnership, however, there is equality in the relationship. The literature identifies that there is no consensus as to what is meant by 'family-centred care', but key themes are identified. FCC recognises the role of the family being central to the child's overall well-being and that families are involved in their child's care to the extent that they choose.

Smith et al. state that FCC is *the professional support of the child and family through a process of involvement, participation and partnership underpinned by empowerment and negotiation* (2002, p22). They identify five stages in the continuum of FCC, indicating the increasing level of contributions the parent makes to the child's care (or for older children, the child's contribution) from no involvement, through involvement, participation, partnership and finally to parent-led care. However, recognising the child as being a partner in their own care, the last stage should be parent/child-led care as appropriate. The five stages (adapted from Smith et al., 2002) are:

1. no involvement: nurse-led;
2. involvement: nurse-led;
3. participation: nurse-led;
4. partnership: equal status;
5. parent-led or child-led.

So long as the parent or child decides where they sit on the continuum, you will be practising FCC. You also need to acknowledge that parents and children may move along the continuum depending on the family situation, or challenges to the family system.

Case study

Lyn and Paul have three children, Jenny aged 12, Philip aged 10, and Joe aged 3½. Joe has Down's syndrome and is awaiting cardiac surgery for a ventricular septum defect. He also has feeding difficulties due to a stricture and has been in hospital for numerous oesophageal stretches to help his swallowing. Lyn has always stayed with him. He started nursery school for half-days and it took a long time for him to settle; for most of the first term Lyn had to leave him at nursery, even though he was extremely distressed.

Paul's mother also lives with the family. She moved in just after her husband died six years ago and was a great help to Lyn and Paul after Joe was born, especially as Paul works away. However, two years ago she was

continued opposite . . .

continued . . .

diagnosed with dementia, which is deteriorating, and she can only be left for very short periods before she becomes disorientated and frightened. Joe's surgery is today; Lyn arrives on the ward obviously anxious and says she cannot be resident with Joe this time. The nurse tells her that Joe needs her to be with him as this will reduce his anxiety and the effects of hospitalisation. Lyn says that she knows this, and will try to be there for Joe. While on the ward she has a phone call from Jenny, her 12 year old, who has been looking after Gran, to say that she needs to get back to school as she has an exam that afternoon.

Activity 5.8   *Decision making*

Read the case study above and answer these questions.

* How do you think Lyn feels?
* What are the factors that are influencing her decisions?
* How do you think Joe's siblings feel?
* How would you manage this assessment in your role as a student nurse?

Outline answers are given at the end of the chapter.

It is very easy to structure FCC around the child and family without considering other demands on that family. Lyn is a mother to three children, one of whom has significant additional healthcare needs; some of these have the potential to be life-limiting and others are lifelong. It is well known that carers worry about what will happen to a child with a disability when they are no longer living. Additionally, there may be an expectation that Jenny and Philip will take over the role of carer to Joe when Lyn and Paul can no longer fulfil that role. This may be an expectation of Lyn and Paul, or one held by Jenny and Philip, even if Lyn and Paul make it clear that Joe is their responsibility. Lyn may be inadvertently confirming the role of family in delivering care as an important value and belief system by the fact that she is also a carer for Paul's mother and Jenny is involved in that care. You have already explored some of the issues faced by young carers in Chapter 4.

The case study shows how important it is for nurses to consider the whole family in a situation like this. While we know it is important for a parent to stay with Joe, it is also important that pressure, however subtle, is not placed on Lyn, as she is in a no-win situation here. While this is a children's ward, it does not mean that children's nurses cannot liaise with adult services to offer extra help towards providing care for Gran while Joe is in hospital, just as we would expect adult service provision to consider and involve children's services when there are children within a family delivering care to an adult. Liaison with Jenny's school, so that they know she is a carer, would also benefit the family, so that Jenny can help with care provision while not falling behind with her school work or being penalised for late arrival.

So FCC provides a framework in which the level of parental and child involvement in the care decisions and delivery is agreed. This is a fluid, not static position, as needs and resources within a family change with time and circumstances, and as other demands are made on the family structure.

Safeguarding

Safeguarding children

This is an area of care that continues to cause anxiety for the professionals involved. The principles of FCC continue even where there are concerns about the standard of care. The Children Act 1989 states that parents want what is best for their child and more recent policy documents have defined that good parenting:

> *involves caring for children's basic needs, keeping them safe and protected, being attentive and showing them warmth and love, encouraging them to express their views and consistently taking these views into account, and providing the stimulation needed for their development and to help them achieve their potential, within a stable environment where they experience consistent guidance and boundaries.*
>
> (HM Government, 2010, pp29–30)

Every Child Matters (DCSF, 2003) identifies the five outcomes fundamental to a child's welfare and development. These are that they have a right to:

*   be healthy;
*   stay safe;
*   enjoy and achieve;
*   make a positive contribution;
*   achieve economic well-being.

Parents who need help should be encouraged to view asking for help as a responsibility rather than as a failure (as we saw in the previous case study). *Every Child Matters* also states:

> *Such intervention should – provided this is consistent with the safety and welfare of the child – support families in making their own plans for the welfare and protection of their children.*
>
> (HM Government, 2010, p30)

Everyone must work collaboratively to ensure the safety of the child, while working with the family to bring about changes in behaviour that will provide the child with the elements of care that are missing, or to provide an environment considered safe. That may mean the removal of the person doing harm to the child, as in cases of sexual abuse.

There are parallels between the way partnership happens and the way change happens. When exploring change theory, we find that people cannot change unless they know what they need to change and what they are aiming for: we say they must 'own that change'. The same themes apply in developing partnerships, because we have to work together with families to facilitate change. However, as explored here and in previous chapters, partnership involves equality. Can there be equality in a relationship where you and other professionals such as doctors and social workers have decided what that change must be, and are also monitoring to ensure compliance with that change plan? The parents are part of this partnership, but know that, if they do not do what is asked of them, the end result may be the removal of the child.

The latest policy document, *Working Together to Safeguard Children*, once again reiterates good practice:

> *The importance of developing a co-operative working relationship is emphasised so that parents or caregivers feel respected and informed; they believe staff are being open and honest with them and in turn they are confident about providing vital information about their child, themselves and their circumstances . . . Similarly, decisions should also be made with their agreement, whenever possible, unless to do so would place the child at risk of suffering significant harm.*
> (HM Government, 2010, p135)

An important caveat here is that, should close working with the family put the child at risk of significant harm, then work can be undertaken without the parent's knowledge or consent; but this is not a get-out clause that professionals can use to avoid working in partnership in safeguarding situations. However, achieving change within a family is more difficult if we are working against them rather than with them.

Safeguarding vulnerable adults

Unlike the safeguarding of children, there is no specific legislation on safeguarding vulnerable adults in England and Wales, although there is in Scotland. The argument is that abuse involving adults, such as physical or sexual abuse, or financial fraud, is already covered within current legislation. This assumes that all adults are able to protect or stand up for themselves, and when they are not able, because of mental health or disability issues, they would be identified as vulnerable. This may not always be the case. When we become aware of adults receiving care from family or friends, we are professionally responsible for assessing whether there are issues of safeguarding that need addressing (Robbins et al., 2009). It is a requirement that all health providers have a developed policy on safeguarding vulnerable adults.

Activity 5.9   *Team working*

- Read your local policy on safeguarding vulnerable adults.
- Identify your role in this issue as a student nurse or registered nurse.

This is for individual reflection and no outline answer is provided.

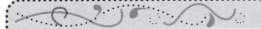

Chapter summary

In this chapter we have explored the concept of family-centred care by examining first the idea of attachment and how it affects children in hospital. We have looked at the concept of a family and how family ties affect the way people cope with illness, especially the way

continued overleaf . . .

continued . . .

they relate to nurses and other health professionals. In terms of assessment, we have discussed how nurses need to find out from carers how much they want to be involved in caring for their loved one in a clinical setting, and we have seen that carers often have multiple roles. There is a continuum of family-centred care, ranging from there being no involvement from the family to it being parent- or child-led, and it should be the family's decision where they are along this continuum. Lastly, we looked at the issues of safeguarding both children and vulnerable adults and the role of the nurse within this.

Activities: brief outline answers

Activity 5.2 Ecomap of family support (page 80)

This is an example of an ecomap.

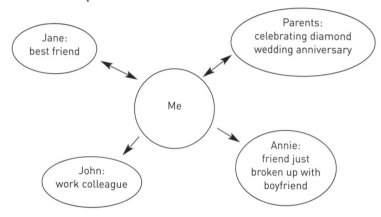

Activity 5.3 An ecomap of a family (page 81)

You need to understand what type of support is offered and how frequently it is given so that your care plan fills the gaps, supports and strengthens the support network, to reduce the chance of it failing. Care from support networks can include the following.

- **Social care**: doing the shopping, clothes washing, walking the dog, paying bills, social conversation, taking the person out for visits and appointments.
- **Physical care**: simple things such as helping with tasks the person is unable to do (putting on socks, applying cream to legs, helping to get dressed, through to undertaking intimate care).
- **Emotional support**: offering the opportunity for the person to chat through worries or concerns.

For this family we need to maximise the mum's potential to successfully breastfeed the baby; we know that stress hormones inhibit milk production and partner support is crucial to success. Gain an understanding of the support mechanisms and use the most supportive – find out what support mum is giving to her mother (the grandmother to the baby); can someone else do this (may need additional professional support here) so that the grandmother can continue to support the family but not take from the family? Offer strategies to reduce stress from the neighbour (we can't solve this but better coping mechanisms can reduce stress). Try to strengthen the support the mum gets from the ante-natal group. Could we change the flow of support from the sister-in-law to supporting the family, rather than taking support from the family until feeding is established?

This is not an exhaustive list by any means.

Activity 5.5 Ben's experience of hospital (page 83)

Ben may be feeling frightened, anxious, scared, lost, alone or abandoned. As Ben's nurse, you might find out these things about him.

- How does he demonstrate anxiety/distress: is it through crying or by becoming very quiet and withdrawn?
- What do his parents do to reassure/comfort him?
- What does he use as a comforter (e.g. teddy, rag doll, blanket)?
- What is Ben's normal routine so that it can be replicated by the nurses to provide continuity for the child?
- What does Ben like to do; what is his favourite game or book? Distraction is a good way to help move the child's focus on to more pleasant activities, but it does not remove pain or discomfort; it is not an alternative to pain relief, but it complements pain relief.

Activity 5.6 Janet and Sean (page 84)

We should be working in partnership with Janet; in the example, this would involve Janet becoming involved in care delivery (participation) at a level she is comfortable with.

Janet may be feeling bad about her role as a mother.

- She may be questioning whether she is a good mum.
- She may feel guilt, as she may believe that she did or didn't do something and that is why Sean is premature.
- She may experience anger/frustration that the birth was very different from how she wanted it to be.
- She may be fearful of all the technology.
- She may be worried that the nurses will judge her by her lack of skills and ability to be involved in his care, even normal baby care – this feeling that the nurses consider her to lack skills may be confirmed to her by the fact that his care is all done by the time she arrives.
- She may feel pressured into engaging in care delivery she has no confidence in because she is worried that she will be judged.

The nurses looking after Sean also have views.

- They may understand her fears and that is why they perform all Sean's care before she gets there.
- They may understand that she has other responsibilities at home and may be trying to reduce demands on her in the hospital.
- They may need to get his care delivered by a certain time to fit in with other treatment demands.
- Nurses need to communicate with Janet to find out how she is feeling and to find out which aspects of his care she wants to engage in.
- Nurses should explain what is being done to Sean and when it needs to be done, so Janet can organise when she is on the ward, if that is what she wants to do.
- They should take time to show Janet how to deliver care to a pre-term infant and help her deliver that care, by giving her support and encouragement as she engages with the care delivery.

Activity 5.8 Lyn and her family (page 87)

Lyn may feel confused, and torn between her various responsibilities. She may feel exhausted physically and mentally by her different roles and the pressure to meet the different demands on her.

The factors that are influencing her decisions might include:

- recognition that, while Joe needs her, he is in a safe environment where nurses will provide for his needs;
- worry that Jenny may not cope with Gran on her own;
- recognition that Jenny's school work is suffering because Lyn is leaving Jenny to provide care for Gran.

Joe's siblings may feel worried about Joe; they may feel proud that they are helping the family and Jenny may feel glad she can reduce some of the burden her mum has in looking after Joe and Gran. Jenny may feel torn between looking after her Gran and needing to be at school. She may feel overwhelmed by the responsibility placed on her; alternatively, she may feel confident in her care skills. Jenny may feel resentment at being a carer for Gran, or she may not recognise she is a carer as it is just part of what families do for each other.

In your role as a student nurse, you need to communicate with Lyn to find out why she can't be there all the time with Joe. Once you know that there is an adult at home who needs care, you should offer Lyn an assessment so that she can access other services to help provide care for Gran, such as referral to the hospital social worker. Agree strategies to use when Lyn is not there in order to reduce Joe's anxiety while in hospital – for example, ask Lynn to leave something for Joe to look after so that he knows she is coming back; use recordings of Lyn's voice to calm Joe; or use Joe's normal comforter, favourite game, song or story. Try to arrange the off duty time so that Joe has a consistent carer, or the least number of nurses involved in his care, so that you provide some continuity for Joe when Lyn isn't there.

Further reading

Moore, L and Kirk, S (2010) A literature review of children's and young people's participation in decisions relating to health care. *Journal of Clinical Nursing*, 19: 2215–25.

This article reviews previous studies on the extent to which children and young people are involved in decision making, the degree of involvement and the types of decisions they are involved in.

National Institute for Health and Clinical Excellence (NICE) (2009) *When to Suspect Child Maltreatment* (Clinical guideline 89). Available online at http://guidance.nice.org.uk/CG89 (accessed 7 February 2011).

This information guide is for anyone involved with children. It outlines the types of signs and symptoms that raise concern and who to report these to.

Rempel, GR, Neufeld, A and Kushner, KE (2007) Interactive use of genograms and ecomaps in family caregiving research. *Journal of Family Nursing*, 13: 403–19.

This article outlines how healthcare staff can utilise genograms and ecopmaps to further knowledge about the family and its relationships and use that information to plan care.

Useful websites

www.actionforsickchildren.org

Action for Sick Children contains information for professionals and families on important child health issues.

www.education.gov.uk

Here you can access the 2006 document, *What To Do If You're Worried a Child is Being Abused*. The Department for Education also contains information for professionals, charities, families and children on a variety of issues relating to child protection at **www.education.gov.uk/schools/pupilsupport/pastoral care/childprotection**.

www.ipfcc.org

The Institute for Patient- and Family-Centered Care is an American site providing information to professionals and families to advance the understanding and practice of patient- and family-centred care in hospitals and other healthcare settings.

Chapter 6
The biographical approach and assessment

NMC Standards for Pre-registration Nursing Education

This chapter will address the following competencies:

Domain 1: Professional values

4. All nurses must work in partnership with service users, carers, families, groups, communities and organisations. They must manage risk, and promote health and wellbeing while aiming to empower choices that promote self-care and safety.
8. All nurses must practice independently, recognising the limits of their competence. They must reflect on these limits and seek advice from, or refer to, other professionals where necessary.

Domain 2: Communication and interpersonal skills

1. All nurses must build partnerships and therapeutic relationships through safe, effective and non-discriminatory communication. They must take account of individual differences, capabilities and needs.
3. All nurses must use verbal, non-verbal and written communication to listen, recognise, interpret and record people's knowledge and understanding of their needs. They must be aware of their own values and beliefs and the impact this may have on their communication with others. They must take account of the many different ways in which people communicate and how these may be influenced by ill health, disability and other factors, and be able to recognise and respond effectively when a person finds it hard to communicate.
8. All nurses must respect individual rights to confidentiality and keep information secure and confidential in accordance with the law and relevant ethical and regulatory frameworks, taking account of local protocols.

Domain 3: Nursing practice and decision-making

1. All nurses must use up-to-date knowledge and evidence to assess, plan, deliver and evaluate care, communicate findings, influence change and promote health and best practice. They must make person-centred, evidence-based judgements and decisions, in partnership with others involved in the care process, to ensure high quality care.
3. All nurses must carry out comprehensive, systematic nursing assessments that take account of relevant physical, social, cultural, psychological, spiritual, genetic and environmental factors in partnership with service users and others through interaction, observation and measurement.

NMC Essential Skills Clusters

This chapter will address the following ESCs:

Cluster: Care, compassion and communication

1. As partners in the care process, people can trust a newly registered graduate nurse to provide collaborative care based on the highest standards, knowledge and competence.

By the first progression point:

2. Works within limitations of the role and recognises own level of competence.
5. Is able to engage with people and build caring professional relationships.

By the second progression point:

6. Forms appropriate and constructive professional relationships with families and other carers.

By entry to the register:

12. Recognises and acts to overcome barriers in developing effective relationships with service users and carers.

2. People can trust the newly registered graduate nurse to engage in person centred care, empowering people to make choices about how their needs are met when they are unable to meet them for themselves.

By the second progression point:

2. Actively empowers people to be involved in the assessment and care planning process.

By entry to the register:

8. Is sensitive and empowers people to meet their own needs and make choices and considers with the person and their carer(s) their capability to care.

5. People can trust the newly registered, graduate nurse to engage with them in a warm, sensitive and compassionate way.

By the first progression point:

4. Provides person centred care that addresses both physical and emotional needs and preferences.

By entry to the register:

8. Listens to, watches for, and responds to verbal and non-verbal cues.
9. Engages with people in the planning and provision of care that recognises personalised needs and provides practical and emotional support.

Introduction

To understand a man, you must first understand his memories.
(Ancient proverb)

As suggested in the proverb, looking at a person's memories helps you to understand that individual. In this chapter we will examine the biographical approach to patients, which is a way of knowing and understanding the patient in greater depth by looking at their life experiences. This can help us to appreciate the patient's perspective and to assess the degree of participation and/or partnership they are looking for in their care. We have seen in previous chapters how this varies among people. Next, we will explore the process of assessment to help you develop your skills in promoting patient and carer involvement in decision-making.

Knowing the patient

Case study

Joan Smith was a 90-year-old lady who had been transferred to a nursing home to convalesce following surgery for a fractured hip, which she had sustained in a fall. She had been finding it increasingly difficult to manage on her own and, following surgery, she was more confused and slow to recover. She had suffered from depression all her adult life. On assessment on admission to the home, her problems were identified as:

- *incontinence of urine and occasionally faeces;*
- *poor appetite;*
- *limited mobility;*
- *confusion;*
- *low mood.*

continued overleaf . . .

continued . . .

> *Four weeks after admission, Joan Smith died. After her death, the following obituary appeared in the local paper:*
>
> Smith, Joan, aged 90, died peacefully in her sleep at Bank Nursing Home. Beloved wife, mother and grandmother. Doctor of philosophy, a lecturer for many years, Justice of the Peace and centre of her community. She was also an artist, lover of music and Bible smuggler.

The staff at the nursing home were shocked to read about 'the real Joan' and realised that they had never got to know her. Have you ever stopped to ask yourself whether you really knew the patient and/or family in your care? The importance of this knowing has emerged as a central concept in nursing, and is the main way that care can be individualised (Radwin, 1996). Radwin's study also concluded that knowing the patient had these two main components:

- the nurse's understanding of the patient;
- selecting individualised interventions.

The first stage in relationship-building is *getting to know the patient which was viewed as essential to achieving the best outcome for the patient* (Luker et al., 2000, p776). This may seem quite obvious, but a busy nurse does not always see this as one of the aims of assessment. Yet it is an essential precursor to the provision of good-quality care (Luker et al., 2000). Little attention had been paid to extending this to the nurse's relationship with family or carers. An action research study of nurses by Manley et al. (2005) looked at what constituted nursing expertise and, from this, they developed a conceptual model. One of the five key components was *knowing the patient*. According to them, *knowing the patient* is about:

- *respect for people and their own view of the world;*
- *respecting patients' unique perspective on their illness / situation;*
- *willingness to promote and maintain a person's dignity at all times;*
- *conscious use of self to promote a helping relationship;*
- *promoting the patient's own decision making;*
- *willingness to relinquish 'control' to the patient;*
- *recognising the patient's / other's expertise.*

(Manley et al., 2005, p23)

If these were turned into questions about your practice, how many would you be able to agree with and which do you need to work on? Perhaps what is most significant about this definition of 'knowing the patient' is that patients, families and carers were involved in the research that developed them. These statements are excellent goals to work towards, and by the use of reflection you may chart your progress towards reaching them.

Apart from knowing the patient, what other kinds of knowing are important for the nurse when taking this approach? It is this question we will look at now.

Required knowledge

In order to know your patient, you need three different types of knowledge (Liaschenko and Fisher, 1999, cited in Stein-Parbury, 2009, pp7–8). They are case knowledge, patient knowledge and person knowledge. Let's look at each of these types of knowledge in turn.

- *Case knowledge* – this is the objective knowledge of the patient's situation, such as the anatomy, physiology and pharmacology. It is the physical disease processes and the type of knowledge that is generalised rather than patient-specific. This means that you can have an understanding of the patient's problem, e.g. appendicitis, without having met the patient. You know the signs and symptoms, the statistics and the treatment.
- *Patient knowledge* – this knowledge is about how individuals are responding to their health situation and requires the nurse to use interpersonal skills in interaction with the patient in order to gain this understanding.
- *Person knowledge* – this is about knowing the patient as a unique individual and what makes them react the way they do. It involves knowing the patient's personal and private biography. It is about why their actions work for them.

Activity 6.1 *Reflection*

Think about a patient you have recently nursed and reflect on their care.

- Can you identify the three types of knowledge or do you struggle with person knowledge?

To assist your reflection, there is an example at the end of the chapter.

The biographical approach to knowing the patient

One of the main elements in the process of caring is *knowing*. This can be defined as *knowing to understand an event as it had meaning in the life of the patient* (Swanson, 1991, p163). To achieve this understanding, you need to appreciate the biographical context of the patient. What and where has he or she been? What has the patient done, and seen? How do the patient's life experiences affect who he or she is now? You need to see issues from the perspective of people who have lived through different eras and in different countries, cultures and so on. While this may seem relevant only to the elderly, family values will also be influenced by these experiences and, therefore, it is also important for family-centred care. To help you consider this, try Activity 6.2.

Activity 6.2 — *Critical thinking*

Think about how different generations might view:

- communism;
- the NHS;
- the information technology explosion of the 1990s.

What would you think of these if you were born in 1925, 1955 or 1985?

Some suggestions are made at the end of the chapter.

The outline answer shows possible different perspectives but, of course, generalisations and assumptions should not be made as each generation comprises very different individuals. However, this activity was about encouraging you to appreciate how life experiences influence your values and beliefs. Healthcare systems in some eastern European countries still reflect their communist past by seeing patients as numbers rather than individuals. Having joined the EU, many people from these countries now live in the UK, and you need to look out for cultural differences. These issues come first; indeed, *questions of fact take second place to understanding the individual's unique and changing perspective as it is mediated by the social context* (Miller, 2000, pxii). It has also been said that *old age, like any other age, is the summation of events and experiences which occur during one's lifetime. Each individual has a unique life history* (Hinchliff et al., 1998, p663). To understand an individual you need to be able to understand them in the context of their history and life events. A useful way of approaching an individual's history is through three key areas (Adams, 1991, cited in Hinchliff et al., 1998, p663).

- Public events such as 9/11. Although these may not impact directly on an individual, they do stand out. For example, you may hear people relating what they were doing or where they were when they heard about 9/11.
- Personal milestones. Everyone has these; some may have more than others and some may be of greater magnitude than others, but we all have a first day at school, getting a job, our first partner.
- Personal memories that are special to the person, for whom they have their own meaning. Explaining why these are special may be difficult, just as returning to an event may lead the individual to place a different interpretation on it. This may also change over time.

Hinchliff et al. (1998) also pointed out that our culture, background and life experiences also shape our beliefs and values, which in turn will affect our health behaviour. You need to understand a patient's life history in order to understand their beliefs and values. You may like to consider this on a personal level by undertaking Activity 6.3.

Activity 6.3   *Reflection*

Draw your own timeline life review. Start with the here and now and work backwards.

- What personal memories do you have of public events?
- What are your personal milestones?
- Note any special social and family events.
- Do you have any special photos or memorabilia?
- What is your earliest memory?
- What personal memories do you cherish?

This is for individual reflection and no outline answer is provided.

Some nurses work with patients suffering from dementia in constructing personal timelines; it is a useful way in which to understand the patient's history and also a stimulating experience for the patient. A biographical approach of this kind offers a broader picture of the individual and a *sense of totality of a life* (Miller, 2000, p8). People's histories can be viewed at two levels: on one level, each individual has their own history with its inherent personal development and changes during their lifespan; on another level, there are the historical events and social change that would impact on this, so that each person has their own unique life history (Miller, 2000). From this it can be seen how people's definition of themselves is central to their being and, therefore, important for you to appreciate if you want to truly understand the individual. People's lived experience will impact on their behaviour and their health choices, and their experience of health and illness. To enable them to maximise their health, you need to empathise with their perspective of the situation by understanding their history.

In clinical practice in some areas, you may have seen the use of treasure boxes or person-centred scrapbooks. These stories can be recorded in the life storybook by the patients themselves, their family/carers or ward staff (Clarke et al., 2003) and in this way the person's life with its important events can be communicated to others. This is particularly important when the patient is unconscious or has dementia, and can no longer discuss such events with you. It may explain behaviour, such as repeated attempts to sweep and clean, if you are aware that the patient was in service during the early part of their life. Adopting a biographical approach should also help you to understand those people who are significant in a patient's life. The use of these biographical approaches enhances relationships between staff and family carers (Clarke et al., 2003). Now we have looked at some of the practical ways that the biographical approach works in nursing, let us turn to the start of the process, in the assessment of the patient.

Assessment

When you only have limited contact with a patient, developing a biographical approach may not always be feasible or relevant. In hospital short-stay areas, for example, you may not have the opportunity to take this approach. However, assessment is central to promoting patient partnership in all clinical areas. Assessment *is the first stage of the nursing process and forms the foundation of all care to follow* (Sully and Dallas, 2005, p74). Unfortunately, assessment is often viewed as just an admission procedure, while it should be more than this (Walsh, 1998). The initial patient assessment has consequences for the subsequent nurse–patient relationship, and also for consultations with other healthcare professionals (Jones and Collins, 2007). It also offers patients the opportunity to discuss with a nurse issues that they might not raise with the doctor.

So your initial assessment of the patient is a starting point of care and is significant in promoting patient participation. It offers you the opportunity to open a participatory relationship with patients and carers, and allows you to assess what level of participation a patient seeks. It must also be comprehensive if subsequent care is not to be flawed by omission: if you do not identify a patient concern, care cannot be directed to meet this need. Your assessment must be an ongoing activity so that it reflects a patient's changing health status (Walsh, 1998; Roper et al., 2000) and possible changes in a patient's desired level of participation. Your assessment is not a one-off activity, but should be a continuous part of nurse–patient interaction.

In the first part of this chapter we looked at three different kinds of knowledge: case, patient and person knowledge (Liaschenko and Fischer, cited in Stein-Parbury, 2009). All of these elements are important in the assessment carried out by nurses. The focus of a nurse's patient assessment is different from that of medical assessment in that nurses are looking for a patient response rather than just at the disease and pathology itself. So assessment is complex and you need to develop your knowledge and understanding of the assessment process and the associated skills. Think about these in Activity 6.4.

Activity 6.4 — *Critical thinking*

You have made an appointment to open a savings account at a building society. On your arrival, the manager shows you to a desk in the corner of the open-plan office and invites you to sit down. She offers you a cup of coffee. Then she asks you a number of questions about your financial status, which she says are to help her to find you the best product. During the conversation, she taps your responses into the computer. At one point, she is interrupted for several minutes by a colleague with a query and temporarily leaves you while she deals with it.

- What do you think the manager does well at this meeting, and why?
- What areas could be improved?
- Would you want to continue to use this building society?

Some suggestions are given at the end of the chapter.

Factors influencing assessment

In transferring the conclusions of Activity 6.4 to nursing, we can see the importance of relationship initiation and first impressions. Interruptions during assessment may make the patient and/or their carer feel devalued in that they do not have your undivided attention (Walker and

Dewar, 2001). Also, if the interaction seemed controlled by the documentation, the individual may feel that they have to fit into the designated boxes on the form. This reduces the quality of data gathered. It is important to treat people as individuals and listen to what they are saying without being distracted. It is difficult when you first start assessing not to be form-bound, and fear of omission may make you focus on this at the expense of listening to the patient. Be careful not to let assessment become a 'box-ticking exercise' (Walsh, 1998). Try using time at the beginning and end of the interaction to allow the patient to discuss their feelings and to raise any concerns (Jones and Collins, 2007). Observe how experienced nurses conduct assessments with patients and try to develop a style that is more conversational and allows time for the patient or carer to respond.

It is also important during assessment to check patient understanding. Try starting with an open question to gauge this, such as 'How do you feel about coming into hospital?' Although nursing assessment is about patient response, it is essential to check their understanding of their medical diagnosis as there may be misunderstandings or questions they did not raise with the medical staff. Consider the following case study.

Case study

Mary, a first-year student nurse, was admitting Mr Jones from the Accident and Emergency Department. When she asked him what he had come in with, he said piles. *As she did not know how to spell the medical term for this,* haemorrhoids, *she called her mentor over to ask how this was done. Her mentor looked at Mr Jones's A & E card and saw that he was being admitted with a* pilonidal sinus. *This is quite different from what Mr Jones thought he had. He had never heard of pilonidal sinus, but had heard of piles and, therefore, thought this was his problem.*

This case study demonstrates how patients do not always query what they do not understand or may have heard incorrectly. Anxiety makes it more likely that we misunderstand things. Also, patients may have been given one medical term and be confused if a different term with the same meaning is used. It is important not to confuse patients with jargon (Walsh, 1998; Timonen and Sihvonen, 2000). So do think about the language you use; medical terminology soon becomes very familiar to you and it is easy to lose sight of the fact that these are strange terms for patients and carers. Also, think about whether you ever try to discourage patients and carers from asking questions; nurses sometimes do this because they are worried patients will ask something they do not know (Jones and Collins, 2007). If a patient or carer asks something you do not know, explain that you are unsure but that you will find out, or will arrange for them to speak to someone, such as your mentor, who does know the answer.

Environment

The environment in which assessment takes place will impact on the quality of interaction. In their own homes, patients will feel in control of the environment and you will be the visitor, but in hospital they may be anxious and also worry about the lack of privacy. In the community, patients can feel inhibited by the presence of other patients; in one study, two-thirds of patients said they did not want their next of kin present during reporting sessions (Timonen and Sihvonen, 2000). You are probably aware that screens do not provide auditory privacy and, therefore, where possible, you should talk to patients somewhere more private. Remember what was discussed in Chapter 4 about confidentiality. This can be a problem if the patient does not speak English and you need an interpreter. You should always try to use the interpreter services available rather than a family member, which can put relationships under strain and also may prevent the patient from disclosing information. If you are unsure how to access interpreter services in your clinical area, ask your mentor to show you. Using an interpreter makes the interaction more difficult and less spontaneous, but there may be no alternative.

Think about your physical position in relation to the patient, especially if they are in bed on admission. This tends to disempower patients during the admission assessment, as you might find in Activity 6.5.

Activity 6.5   *Communication*

Ask a friend to participate in this activity.

- In turn, one of you should lie on the floor while the other remains standing and asks questions about what you did the previous evening.
- Reverse roles.
- Discuss what feelings were generated by being in each position.

An outline answer is given at the end of the chapter.

Activity 6.5 may have helped you realise how important your position is in relation to the patient. You will have found it difficult to offer your perspective when lying flat on your back gazing up at your friend, and yet patients often find themselves in this disadvantaged position, and speaking to a stranger. So think how you can adjust your position to reduce this disadvantage to the patient. You need also to remember to bend down to be on a level with children and adopt a position on the same level as someone in a wheelchair.

Consent

Before you make any assessment, you must have consent from the patient. There are three elements in gaining consent, which are *competency, information and voluntariness* (Dougherty and Lister, 2008, p5). Information is fundamental to giving informed consent. Patients and carers need to be told why you want information from them, and what is the purpose of the assessment, so that they feel comfortable about divulging personal information. Think back to Activity 6.4 (on page 100) and how you might wonder why you were being asked some of the questions. To consider competency and voluntariness, see the 'Further reading' at the end of the chapter.

Assessment skills

You will need a variety of skills to perform patient assessment. The key ones are:

- interpersonal skills;
- observational skills;
- measurement;
- physical examination.

The latter two skills will vary according to the field of nursing, but observational and inter-personal skills are used throughout nursing and it is these we will now look at.

Way back in 1859 Florence Nightingale herself stated that observation was the most important lesson for nurses, and even suggested that nurses should cease nursing if they could not learn to be observant! More recently, observation has been described as *a high level skill that requires a great deal of practice* (Murray and Atkinson, 2000, p34), and nurses have said that they gained much valuable information about patients by *just looking* (Latimer, 2000, p103). Observation is also important for picking up discrepancies between verbal and non-verbal communication, in which case the latter is generally more reliable. Some nursing students are naturally more observant than others, but it is an essential skill in assessment. To illustrate how much information can be gained this way, try Activity 6.6.

Activity 6.6   *Critical thinking*

Use the body outline below to note what information can be gained by observation.

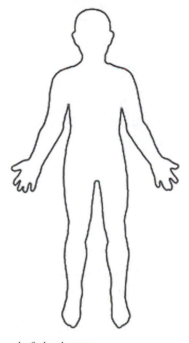

An outline answer is given at the end of the chapter.

If you feel that your observational skills need improving, set yourself daily challenges in clinical practice. At breaks, try to think back to your group of patients and state what colour clothing they were wearing. Who wears glasses? If you are in a hospital, what was on their lockers? Set yourself these types of questions and then, after your break, check out your answers. Prior to assessment, make sure that, if a patient uses a hearing aid or glasses, they have these and that they are working. Think how frustrating it is when you cannot quite hear a television programme because the sound is turned down. To promote partnership, both parties must have equal opportunity to participate, and this is never more so than at this crucial initial assessment.

Your interpersonal skills will be developing throughout your education and there is 'Further reading' recommended for this. One of the key areas to consider in assessment is the type of questions asked, and we will look at this in the next activity.

Activity 6.7　　　　　　　　　　　　　　　　　　　*Communication*

Match the questions (a–g) to the types of questions (1–7) and think of one or two of your own examples.

1. **Closed**, which have limited answers. They can be used for checking factual information or when someone is breathless or has difficulty speaking.
2. **Open**, which offer the opportunity to say what you want.
3. **Recall**, which are about recounting experience.
4. **Affective**, which are about feelings.
5. **Rhetorical**, which answer themselves and should not be used.
6. **Leading**, which suggest what answers should be given.
7. **Accusatory**, which are judgemental.

a. Are you still smoking?
b. Are you working?
c. When did your headaches start?
d. How do you feel about your operation?
e. What can you tell me about your family?
f. You think that this is a nice room, don't you?
g. Who wouldn't be upset by that?

Answers are given at the end of the chapter.

You should not be using the last three types of questions. Observe how your mentor asks questions and think how you use them. At first, it is easy to be driven by questions that arise from the documentation that you are required to complete for admission, but remember that this can result in an interview that sounds like an interrogation. Experienced nurses will be able to have a more open conversation, which gently introduces the topics that need to be covered. However, do remember to allow space for the patient and/or carer to think about their answers and give them time to follow their own agenda. The following research summary highlights some key points about nursing assessment.

Research summary: 'Nursing assessments and other tasks: influences on participation in interactions between patients and nurses' (Jones and Collins, 2007)

Aim: to explore nursing assessment and highlight factors that influence patient participation and factors that enhance communication.

Data collection: 49 video-/audio-taped nurse–patient encounters in three different settings – 27 admission interviews in a general hospital ward, 19 review meetings for diabetic patients in general practice, and three specialist cancer nurse head and neck consultations in outpatients. Total of 53 patients involved.

Findings: predominant feature was question–answer format of interviews. Patient contribution in the encounter was found to be correlated to the nurse's organisation and prioritisation of topics.

Factors restricting participation: being task bound; the documentation and the writing of responses reduced the nurses' sensitivity to patients' expressions of concern. When patients did raise concerns, these were not explored but cut short and a return made to the document. A recurrent theme was preoccupation with the document over spontaneous communication with the patient.

Factors enhancing communication: positive nurse–patient relationships; time for spontaneous communication.

Recommendations: clearly identify the purpose of the assessment and maximise opportunities for patient contribution by use of open questions. Utilise strategies to encourage patients to pursue their thoughts. Think about the time required or how this could be organised to provide patients with the opportunity to raise issues.

Sources of information

While the primary source of information should be the patient, this may not always be possible if the patient is a young child or unconscious. However, you might also seek information from secondary sources, such as the patient's relatives, friends or significant others, along with medical or nursing records (Hogston and Simpson, 2007). Make sure that the patient feels free to express their perspective and, if a partner or parent is interrupting or taking over, go back and check with the patient when they are on their own. Where the patient is dependent on carers, it is essential that you include the carer perspective.

> ## Case study
>
> *Mrs Smith had come with her 80-year-old mother, who lives with her but needed to go to hospital after a fall. Mrs Smith offered to collect some personal belongings for her mother from home, but the nurse admitting her mother said that it would not be necessary to return with these until the following day as they could provide her mother with enough for the night. Mrs Smith hesitated and said, 'Shall I say goodbye, then?' 'Yes', said the nurse, 'we'll look after your mother now.' Mrs Smith wanted to stay but the nurse seemed to be dismissing her. She wanted to discuss with the nurse how her mother got confused at night and how it was important to do things in the same way she always did. How would the nurses know this, if they did not ask her about her mother's normal activities of daily living?*

The daughter in this case study has valuable information to offer but is dismissed. You may feel when you are assessing a patient that it is easier dealing with just one person, but this will not always provide enough information, and you need to encourage carer participation where appropriate. The following questions suggested by Walker and Dewar (2001) may be helpful to you.

- *What are the priorities and concerns of the nursing/medical staff and the carer with regard to the patient's care?*
- *What should the care plan promote, maintain and prevent in relation to this individual's care?*
- *What action needs to be taken in order to realise this care plan?*
- *What information is needed by both parties to do this?*
- *What support does the carer need? Do they need information about services, such as local carer organisations?*
- *What level of involvement does the carer want?*
- *Are there any constraints on the carer on this involvement?*
- *How will the on-going relationship between carer and practitioners be maintained and evaluated?*

(p335)

These questions should be not be delivered as a checklist or cross-examination, but woven into the conversation. You need to consider when it is more appropriate to talk to the carer and patient separately. If the patient wants to discuss embarrassing or personal information, it may be necessary to ask the carer to leave. Sometimes, the presence of carers or parents can dominate an assessment. In this instance, thank them for their response but persist in ensuring that the patient has the opportunity to answer. The following activity is designed to help you reflect on these issues.

Activity 6.8 — *Reflection*

Think back to an initial patient and/or carer assessment you have recently conducted and write a brief description. You may wish to use a reflective model.

- How did you ensure that the environment was conducive to patient/carer participation?
- Did you introduce yourself and explain the purpose of the assessment?
- How spontaneous was the interaction or were you controlling it by the use of questions?
- What types of questions did you use?
- Did you allow the patient/carer time to respond?
- What observations did you make?
- Did you feel that the interaction was inhibited by your writing of responses?
- Did you allow time for questions, and how comfortable did you feel with this?
- Were there any interruptions?
- How did you feel the nurse–patient relationship was developing in terms of participation/partnership?
- What did you feel you did well?
- What would you do differently another time?

This is for individual reflection and no outline answer is provided.

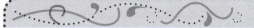

Chapter summary

This chapter has looked at the use of biography to promote understanding of the patient as an individual with a unique life history. Next, we discussed the importance of the assessment process in developing an understanding of the individual and their family/carers. This process is essential in establishing a nurse–patient relationship that promotes participation and partnership. Assessment also establishes what level of participation patients and carers are wanting. The next two chapters will look at how this assessment can be built on to promote participation by encouraging self-management and health literacy.

Activities: brief outline answers

Activity 6.1 Types of knowledge (page 97)

- **Knowing**: Mr Bloggs has just returned from theatre following a transurethral resection of prostate (TURP).
- **Case knowledge**: post-operative care for TURP, which would include monitoring pulse and blood pressure for haemorrhage and shock, fluid balance, catheter care, prevention of deep vein thrombosis, control of pain.

If you only use this level of knowledge, you are nursing using a biomedical model as described in Chapter 1.

- **Patient knowledge**: allergic to penicillin; deaf in left ear; tendency towards constipation (self-medicates for this at home), which may be exacerbated by opiate analgesia and reduced mobility, but needs to avoid straining after pelvic surgery.
- **Person knowledge**: has never married and is worried about female staff undertaking care that involves touching his genitals. This is the first time he has had surgery and he does not know what to expect. He is very frightened because a close friend recently died shortly after surgery.

Activity 6.2 Generational perspectives (page 98)

- **Communism**: those born in 1925 and 1955 remember the Cold War, the Cuban crisis in the 1960s, the arms race, escapes across the Berlin Wall. Still, perhaps, a bit wary of the East. Those born in 1985 were only four when the Wall came down and have little knowledge of what communism meant.
- **NHS**: those born in 1925 remember how, sometimes, you did not go to the doctor before 1948 because you could not afford it, so they are grateful for free treatment and take what is on offer without questioning. Those born in 1955 and 1985 have always known free healthcare and have only heard older relatives talk of 'poor law hospitals'.
- **IT explosion**: those born in 1925 may not have access to nor understand the internet; they may not know how to text. Those born in 1955 have seen the big changes and have strived to keep up with them; they can see the benefits. Those born in 1985 cannot remember life before the internet and could not exist without a mobile phone.

Activity 6.4 Building society appointment (page 100)

- **Good practice**: she is punctual and welcoming; she introduces herself, offers you a drink, offers you a seat, explains the purpose of meeting and listens to you.
- **Privacy**: you may still be overheard and the office may be noisy. Is the office too hot or cold? Did the use of a computer distract you from your responses or did you feel that she was following a script without acknowledging your response? Did you have an opportunity to check what was inserted on to the form? The interruption makes you feel unimportant, as she is wasting your time and putting other people before you.

Activity 6.5 Physical position (page 102)

- **Lying down**: vulnerable, disempowered, obliged to give answers.
- **Standing**: in control, confident, feeling superior.

Activity 6.6 Observational skills (page 103)

- General demeanour, appearance?
- Hair – texture; is it cared for? Alopecia?
- Eyes – expression, protruding, any jaundice, bloodshot, pupils – equal, fixed? False eye?
- Ears – hearing aid?
- Mouth – halitosis, dentures, broken teeth, state of mouth?
- Face – expression, florid, pallor, cyanosis?
- Skin – texture, dryness, rashes, bruises, evidence of self-harm, puncture sites, hydration, varicosities, hirsutism, hydration, operation scars, pressure sores, oedema?
- Fingernails – smoker, nail-biting, anaemia (spoon shaped), clean?
- Chest – depth of respiration, evenness, coughing, wheezing?
- Genitalia – any abnormalities?
- Joints – fixed, swollen?
- Smell – alcohol, vomit, faeces, urine, staining of clothes?
- Clothes – weight loss or gain?

Activity 6.7 Types of question (page 104)

1b; 2e; 3c; 4d; 5f; 6g; 7a.

Further reading

Bach, S and Grant, A (2009) *Communication and Interpersonal Skills for Nurses.* Exeter: Learning Matters.

This is useful for developing your ability to establish therapeutic relationships.

Collins, S, Britten, N, Ruusuvuori, J and Thompson, A (2007) *Patient Participation in Health Care Consultations.* Basingstoke: Open University Press.

Different chapters report studies into patient participation in differing healthcare contexts.

Dougherty, L and Lister, S (eds) (2008) *The Royal Marsden Hospital Manual of Clinical Nursing Procedures.* Oxford: Blackwell Publishing.

See chapters 1, 2 and 3 for further information on consent, assessment and communication.

Lloyd, H and Craig, S (2007) A guide to taking a patient's history. *Nursing Standard*, 22(13): 42–8.

This provides information for structuring a nursing history.

Miller, R (2000) *Researching Life Stories and Family Histories.* London: Sage.

This book contains research studies in the different fields of nursing, conducted using a biographical approach.

Sully, P and Dallas, J (2005) *Essential Communication Skills for Nurses.* Edinburgh: Elsevier Mosby.

Chapter five, on interview and assessment skills, offers further information about factors to consider in the assessment process.

Useful websites

www.culturediversity.org/basic.htm

This site explores Leininger's theory of transcultural nursing. In assessment, you need to be culturally sensitive and this theory may be helpful to you in thinking about the influence of cultural issues on health and communication.

www.nmc-uk.org

Search this site for further guidance on documentation.

Chapter 7
Supporting self-care

NMC Standards for Pre-registration Nursing Education

This chapter will address the following competencies:

Domain 1: Professional values

3. All nurses must support and promote health, wellbeing, rights and dignity of people, groups, communities and populations. These include people whose lives are affected by ill health, disability, ageing, death and dying. Nurses must understand how these activities influence public health.

4. All nurses must work in partnership with service users, carers, families, groups, communities and organisations. They must manage risk, and promote health and wellbeing whilst aiming to empower choices that promote self-care and safety.

5. All nurses must fully understand the nurse's various roles, responsibilities and functions and adapt their practice to meet the changing needs of people, groups, communities and populations.

Domain 2: Communication and interpersonal skills

5. All nurses must use therapeutic principles to engage, maintain and, where appropriate, disengage from professional caring relationships, and must always respect professional boundaries.

6. All nurses must take every opportunity to encourage health-promoting behaviour through education, role modelling and effective communication.

Domain 3: Nursing practice and decision-making

1. All nurses . . . must make person-centred, evidence-based judgements and decisions in partnership with others involved in the care process, to ensure high quality care . . ..

8. All nurses must provide educational support, facilitation skills and therapeutic nursing interventions to optimise health and well-being. They must promote self-care and management whenever possible, helping people to make choices about their healthcare needs, involving families and carers where appropriate to maximise their ability to care for themselves.

NMC Essential Skills Clusters

This chapter will address the following ESCs:

Cluster: Care, compassion and communication

2. People can trust the newly registered graduate nurse to engage in person centred care, empowering people to make choices about how their needs are met when they are unable to meet them for themselves.

By the second progression point:

2. Actively empowers people to be involved in the assessment and care planning process.
4. Actively supports people in their own care and self-care.
5. Considers with the person and their carer their capability for self-care.

By entry to the register:

8. Is sensitive and empowers people to meet their own needs and make choices and considers with the person and their carer(s) their capability to care.
14. Actively helps people to identify and use their strengths to achieve their goals and aspirations.

5. People can trust the newly registered nurse to engage with them in a warm, sensitive and compassionate way.

By the first progression point:

4. Provides person centred care that addresses both physical and emotional needs and preferences.

By entry to the register:

9. Engages with people in the planning and provision of care that recognises personalised needs and provides practical and emotional support.

Cluster: Organisational aspects of care

10. People can trust the newly registered graduate nurse to deliver nursing interventions and evaluate their effectiveness against the agreed assessment and care plan.

By the second progression point:

1. Acts collaboratively with people and their carers enabling and empowering them to take a shared and active role in the delivery and evaluation of nursing interventions.

By entry to the register:

10. Involves the person in review and adjustments to their care, communicating changes to colleagues.

Introduction

Give a person a fish, and you feed him for a day. Teach him how to fish and you feed him for a lifetime.
(Proverb)

This well-known proverb is often quoted by authors writing about self-care, and is useful here to underpin what this chapter is about. The meaning is clear: being given a fish is passive, but being taught how to fish involves active participation. In the previous chapter, we looked at how important it is for you to assess patients and carers as individuals, so as to establish how much they want to participate in their care. In this chapter, we will look at how you can support that participation by promoting self-care and self-management. It begins by looking at the meaning of self-care, and goes on to look at how you can promote self-care with patients and carers.

Self-care

First of all, we need to consider what we mean by self-care. One of the most widely used nursing models over the last part of the twentieth century was one created by Dorothea Orem from her original work in the 1950s (Walsh, 1998). This model, which you may have seen in practice, is based on the assumption that people want to self-care. Orem defines self-care as *an adult's continuous contribution to his or her own continued existence, health and well being* (2001, p44). She goes on to say that it is *action deliberately performed by persons to regulate their own functioning and development or that of their dependants* (p45). If you look at this definition, you will see that self-care activity is seen not only as essential for living, but also as a way of improving the quality of that life by enabling the individual to develop and to enhance their health. Walsh considered that Orem's belief was that *people strive to self care by their own effort and when they cannot, by the efforts of family or significant others* (1998, p115). This last point is important because it may be the carers you will be supporting so that they can provide the necessary care for the patient.

Self-care has been a focus of nursing for quite some time, but has more recently been promoted by the government, with the Department of Health (2005a) producing a very similar definition to Orem's. The Department declared that it was actions that people took for their own health and well-being and also saw that this action might be taken on behalf of others, such as children, family and friends. This action is seen as essential not only to maintain physical and mental health, but also to meet social and psychological needs (DH, 2005a). The NMC has defined self-care as:

> *personal health maintenance. It is any individual, family or community activity that aims to improve or restore health, or treat or prevent disease. It includes all health decisions people make for themselves and their families.*
> (2010, p151)

The Department of Health (2005a) saw self-care as being particularly important for people with long-term health conditions (15.4 million people) and also after discharge from hospital. You may recall from Chapter 4 how carers outlined their need to be involved in care decisions, and this is particularly so when the patient has mental health problems or long-term health conditions:

> *When you leave the clinic, you still have a long-term condition. When the visiting nurse leaves your home, you still have a long-term condition. In the middle of the night, you fight the pain. At the weekend, you manage without your home help.*
> (Cayton, 2005, p2)

Even when you are a nurse working with people in the community, those people have to cope most of the time by themselves. With hospital stays becoming shorter, you have only a short period of time in which to enable people to learn to cope with their health problems. Half of the people in a survey by the Department of Health (2005b) who had seen a healthcare professional in the previous six months stated that they had not been encouraged to self-care, and a third said that they had *never* been encouraged by professionals to do so; but the survey found that people did want to self-care and were looking for more help from professionals. You must remember, however, that self-care is not about professionals just handing over care to patients and carers and leaving them to it; it is about educating, supporting and helping them to do so. The lady who was taught to self-catheterise (see the case study in Chapter 1, on page 7) would have needed much support to enable her to do this.

Self-care policy

The government's drive for self-care is enshrined in the policy that was discussed in Chapter 2. The Department of Health saw self-care as one of the key elements of its drive for patient-centred care, as outlined in the *NHS Improvement Plan*: *It is an important strand to the Government's overall strategy for health* (2005c, p29). It is important that you learn to support patients and carers to self-care. You need, therefore, to think about what self-care means and Activity 7.1 will help you to do this.

Activity 7.1   *Critical thinking*

- Think what self-care activities you have undertaken since you got up this morning.
- Did you perform these unaided?

continued overleaf . . .

continued . . .

- Ask a parent what self-care activities they have carried out for their child.
- Ask an older person or a person with a disability what they have done to self-care.

Some suggestions are given at the end of the chapter.

Activity 7.1 is designed to start you thinking about how diverse and complex self-care can be. The Department of Health (2005a) describes a continuum of complexity, from being able to brush your teeth through to requiring total personal support from a professional. You may well have achieved a range of self-care activities unaided but, equally, if you had a health problem such as diabetes, you would need to take special measures with your eating and drinking, and think about this in relation to physical activity. You would need to be careful with your foot hygiene. The parent may have been teaching their child to self-care, for example tying shoelaces, which, as you may know, can take longer than doing it yourself. It is important to realise this, as promoting patient self-care could be seen as a way of reducing staff time but, in fact, it takes time to educate people and, if done well, can be very time-consuming. You may find in practice that you are tempted to finish off an activity for a patient or carer and think that you are helping, as they may be struggling, but in the longer term, when you are not around, they need to be able to do it unaided. Self-care is about partnership, and promoting patient and carer autonomy.

You will need to negotiate with your patient in order to meet their care needs using a self-care approach (Walsh, 1998). According to the Department of Health, self-care is *about the choices people make and the actions that they take on their own behalf in the interest of maintaining their health and well-being* (2010a, p7). Returning to Activity 7.1, we need to explore this continuum of self-care activities further.

Types of self-care

In Activity 7.1, you may have identified some self-care activities that everyone would perform and some that you would only undertake in a particular context, such as if you had a health problem.

There are three types of self-care requirements, according to Orem (2001):

- **universal**: those types of activities that we all need to carry out in order to live, such as eat, drink and breathe;
- **developmental**: activities we need to perform at certain points in our lives, such as during pregnancy, where we have a need to adjust and to learn about our new situation;
- **health deviation**: self-care needs that arise from having a health condition such as depression, which means that we have to learn how to cope by, for example, learning about medication regimes.

When you are supporting people to self-care, you might be negotiating with people to make healthier choices to meet their universal needs. In meeting developmental needs, you might be engaged with first-time parents in caring for their new baby. Meeting health deviation needs means that you are enabling people to make choices about their care options in order to maximise their health potential.

The Department of Health (2005c) has produced a model for supporting people with long-term conditions, which also identifies differing levels of self-care. Nurses and other health professionals underpin this support by helping people to make healthy lifestyle choices, such as taking more exercise. As a nurse, you are in an ideal position to provide people with information about lifestyle choices and to discuss ways of achieving a healthier lifestyle, as in the following case study.

Case study

Julie was a single mother who had developed post-natal depression after the birth of her first child. She was recovering at home with the support of Rita, the community psychiatric nurse. Rita found Julie a local mother and baby group, which she attended with help. Rita went with Julie and the baby at first, but then Julie managed to go on her own. Rita also talked to Julie about the importance of diet and not neglecting herself. She discussed with Julie ways of affording a diet in line with health recommendations on her limited budget and encouraged her to cook for herself.

The case study demonstrates how nurses who have professional contact with patients should seek to promote healthy lifestyle choices. We can apply the DH model of self-care (2005c, p10) to this case.

- **Supported self-care**: where individuals and their carers develop sufficient knowledge and skills to cope with their condition confidently. This would be about helping Julie to understand her condition and strategies for coping.
- **Disease-specific management**: a multi-disciplinary team approach to meeting the needs of people who have complex needs.
- **Case management approach**: where people require very high-intensity interventions.

The relationship between self-care and self-management

These two terms are sometimes used interchangeably, but whereas self-care includes self-management, self-care is about individual or family responsibility for health and well-being, while self-management is about people making the most of what they have, such as maximising their life potential when they have a health condition (Skills for Care and Skills for Health, 2008). A key feature of self-management is the individual's understanding of their illness and ongoing involvement in their care (Warwick et al., 2010). Self-management has also been defined as *individuals making the most of their lives by coping with difficulties and making the most of what they have* (Skills for Care and Skills for Health, 2008, p9). Self-management education can also be seen as one of a range of interventions, perhaps the best-known intervention coming under the umbrella term of self-care (Coulter and Ellins, 2006). Self-management education, according to these authors, differs from patient education in that the latter is disease-specific information delivered by healthcare professionals who encouraged patients in order to promote compliance, while self-management education is broader and aims to improve self-efficacy. Self-management education might be led by a health professional, but could equally be led by a peer leader or other patients, often in group settings.

In promoting self-care and self-management, you need to adopt a facilitative rather than a didactic approach. Instead of telling patients what to do, you need to help them understand why they need to do it, and show them how. You need to think about working with patients and carers rather than just teaching them about their condition. In self-management education, you need to engage in participatory learning techniques. Nurses are *at the forefront of a national shift towards self-management* (Davies, 2010, p53), so developing these skills is essential.

Requirements for self-care

In this section we will look at what patients need in order to self-care.

Activity 7.2 *Reflection*

Think about all the situations you have read about so far where patients self-care.

- What would a patient need in order to self-care?
- What skills do you as a nurse need to support patients and carers to self-care?

Outline answers are given at the end of the chapter.

These are the ways that nurses support patients in order to self-care:

- *Acting or doing for another.*
- *Guiding and directing.*
- *Providing physical and psychological support.*
- *Providing and maintaining an environment that supports personal development.*
- *Teaching.*

(Orem, 2001, p56)

These are the skills that you need to develop during your education. The Department of Health (2008a) identified four key elements for supporting self-care: information, tools (such as self-monitoring), skills and support networks. Information-giving will be discussed in the next chapter, and is fundamental to patients and carers being able to make informed decisions about their care. Skills development and support networks will be discussed later in this chapter. Self-monitoring could be by technological means, such as the monitoring of blood glucose levels in diabetes. There is a range of technologies for monitoring glucose levels, including DiaBetNet, which is a diabetic monitoring system with an interactive game for teenagers on their mobile phones (DH, 2005d). You need to be familiar with these tools and self-monitoring devices because they are an integral part of assisting people to self-care and take control of their situation (DH, 2008a). When you are nursing patients who use such technology, you should ask yourself the following questions:

- *Do you know what self-monitoring devices and tools people currently use?*
- *Do they know how to use them?*
- *Is there new equipment that might improve their quality of life?*
- *Do you know how individuals might gain access to such equipment?*

(DH, 2008a, p13)

Coulter and Ellins (2006) found that patients with hypertension benefited from being able to self-monitor their own blood pressure, and the same is true for those on anticoagulant therapy. It depends on your field of nursing how much your patients use technology for self-care. For further examples of monitoring and assistive tools, visit **www.dh.gov.uk/selfcare**.

One way in which patients can improve their knowledge and skills is through the Expert Patients Programme (see **www.expertpatients.co.uk**). This is a self-management programme for people living with long-term health conditions. It helps patients develop new skills that enable them to better manage their condition on a day-to-day basis, and we will look at it in some detail now.

Expert patients

Activity 7.3 *Reflection*

- Have you heard about the Expert Patients Programme?
- If you had a long-term condition, such as diabetes, how would you feel about attending such a programme?
- What would you hope to gain from the programme?

Outline answers are given at the end of the chapter.

The first self-management programmes were developed in the UK in the 1990s, with the co-operation of self-help groups such as Arthritis Care, the Manic Depression Fellowship and Changing Faces. The Expert Patients Programme (EPP) was announced in *Saving Lives* (DH, 1999b) as the final strand of the Healthy Citizens initiative. The idea was that people with chronic conditions were in the best place themselves to work out coping strategies, so the Chief Medical Officer set up a task force to examine the possibilities and to design a pilot programme to enable people to improve their self-esteem and quality of life. This resulted in the report, *The Expert Patient: A new approach to chronic disease management for the 21st century* (DH, 2001a), which recommended the establishment of lay-led self-management programmes within the NHS.

A structured programme of self-care skills training is a key mechanism for achieving the goal of increased patient involvement (Rogers, 2009). The EPP is a generic programme whose aim is to improve the quality of life of people with long-term conditions. It seeks to do this by supporting the patient to develop self-care skills, and to build up their confidence and also their motivation to take more control over their life and illness.

The EPP was developed from work undertaken in Stanford, USA, by Kate Lorig and her team (Street and Powell, 2008). They conducted research into the links between patient education and health status. They found that a person's overall state of health was greatly influenced by their emotional state and their feeling of being in control. The Stanford course was open to anyone with a long-term condition, and run by trained volunteers or paid trainers who were licensed to do so (see 'Useful websites' at the end of the chapter). All the evidence suggested that this self-management of chronic conditions could improve health status while reducing hospitalisations. Because it was undertaken in a different healthcare system, this evidence is not transferable. The first EPPs were launched in England and Wales in 2002, under licence from Stanford University, with 26 pilot courses. By the end of the pilot phase in 2004, there were almost 300 courses. *Our Health, Our Care, Our Say* (DH, 2006a) made a commitment to increasing capacity from 12,000 to 100,000 places per year by 2012. This white paper also announced the setting up of a not-for-profit community interest company (EPPCIC) to market and deliver the programme.

Benefits of the programme

Case study

Jo is a divorcee who is 48 years old and has daughters aged 8 and 11. Her marriage had been in difficulties, but when she developed rheumatoid arthritis six years ago it collapsed completely. Jo found the symptoms, particularly the pain, difficult to cope with. Financially, she could just about manage without working but, while the girls were at school, she could not bring herself to do very much. All this dented her self-esteem and she felt very low. Her GP suggested that attending an EPP might help and offer her insights into managing her condition. Jo was sceptical about attending the course at first, but she found it very helpful. She was surprised how much she had in common with her fellows, even though they had different health conditions. She gained new motivation and decided to train as a course coordinator. This boosted her self-esteem and she decided to become involved with nurse education at her local university. Jo found that her health improved so much that, when both her girls were in secondary education, she found paid employment.

Jo's case study demonstrates that finding out that you are not alone, and that there are other people who also experience low self-esteem and pain from their conditions, can be liberating and help the individual to develop self-confidence and self-efficacy (Street and Powell, 2008). The EPP is aimed at people at the first level ('Supported self-care') of the Department of Health model (2005c). It is to encourage those who represent 70–80 per cent of people with long-term health conditions to become active partners in their own care. This programme is *another model of patient-led change created in this case by people with long-term conditions for people with long-term conditions* (Cayton, 2008, p37), and the focus of these programmes is on *personal motivation, decision-making, goal setting, dealing with pain and fatigue and getting the best from health professionals* (ibid.).

The programme should help people not only to be realistic about the impact of their disease on themselves and their family, but also to use their skills and knowledge to lead full lives. In particular, patients should benefit from being able to engage more effectively with healthcare professionals and to work in partnership. As a nurse, you need to know about the EPPs available to patients in your area and field of nursing.

Structure of the Expert Patients Programme

The EPP is a six-week course with once-weekly sessions of two and a half hours. There is a follow-up session, three months after completion. Groups comprise 10–16 participants. Sometimes the course tutors have the long-term condition themselves, and act as role models (Taylor and Bury, 2007, cited in Street and Powell, 2008); it helps participants to see what they might be able to achieve (Cayton, 2008). An online version of the EPP has been developed, and programmes have now been developed by the EPPCIC for young people aged 12–18 and run by young people. The EPPCIC also developed and ran Caring with Confidence, which was a generic programme designed for carers. For more details of all these programmes, see the 'Useful websites' at the end of the chapter.

Activity 7.4   *Communication*

- Do you know if there is an EPP operating in your area?
- As a nurse, what do you feel about the term 'expert patient'?

A outline answer is given at the end of the chapter.

You might feel a bit threatened by the term 'expert', particularly as a student. There is a danger that the term might feel challenging to your professional expertise (Street and Powell, 2008) but these programmes are not designed to impart professional knowledge but to help patients find resources from within themselves (Cayton, 2008). It is only a problem if nurses and other healthcare professionals want to *direct* patients and carers rather than facilitate them to enhance their own health, so you need to reflect on how you would feel if a patient had undertaken such a programme. Patients may well know more than you do but, instead of feeling threatened by this, try to see it as an opportunity to learn from them and to work in partnership.

Evaluation of Expert Patients Programmes

You will be aware that any health intervention needs to be evaluated, and so far the findings about programmes such as this are mixed (Coulter and Ellins, 2006). In 2006, the National Primary Care Research & Development Centre conducted evaluative research into the EPP, using both quantitative and qualitative techniques. Their qualitative findings showed that people reported an increase in self-efficacy. They highly valued the social support offered by the group. Some respondents, however, would have preferred a condition-specific group. The randomised controlled trial found that there were benefits to self-efficacy and self-reported energy levels, but no difference in health service utilisation. The programme was, however, deemed to be cost-effective. There is an issue that some courses have struggled with recruitment and that the initial courses were taken up by people who were already self-managing. White middle-class people were also over-represented. You can bear these findings in mind when patients ask your opinion about such courses.

Disease-specific programmes

There is no doubt that the greatest benefit in self-management for patients comes from EPP courses on specific conditions (Warwick et al., 2010). The availability of these courses will vary with your field of nursing and you need to ask about what applies in your clinical area. Examples of such programmes are Dose Adjustment for Normal Eating (DAFNE) and Diabetes Education and Self Management for Ongoing and Newly Diagnosed (DESMOND). You may find that your local GP practice offers disease-specific groups, but these may be led by a health professional and may not apply the principles of peer support and facilitation of patient self-management of symptoms and medication.

Common Core Principles to Support Self Care

These principles form the basis of a key document (Skills for Care and Skills for Health, 2008) on self-care. Keen and Lewis (2008) have stated that the main purpose of these principles is to facilitate *reflection, challenge and practice change* (p3). They support government policy on the personalisation of health, and are designed to promote partnership working and ensure that people play a central role in their care. They are useful principles for everyone working in health, especially nurses. You need to reflect on these principles and think about how they apply in your practice. Can you see these at work in your practice, and identify any you need to work on?

Research summary: The principles of self-care

1. Ensure that individuals are able to make informed choices to manage their self-care needs.
2. Communicate effectively to enable individuals to assess their needs and develop and gain confidence in self-care.
3. Support and enable individuals to access appropriate information to manage their self-care needs.
4. Support and enable individuals to develop skills in self-care.
5. Support and enable individuals to use technology to support self-care.
6. Advise individuals on how to access support networks and participate in the planning, development and evaluation of services.
7. Support and enable risk management and risk-taking to maximise independence and choice.

In this list, 'individual' is used to include patients, people who use services and carers.

(Source: Skills for Care and Skills for Health, 2008, p13.)

These core principles sum up much of the nursing practice we have discussed earlier in this chapter and in previous chapters. They also reflect the ESCs relating to partnership working. The interpersonal skills that underpin these principles are of central importance and you will need to develop these throughout your nursing career. Further information about what is needed to achieve these principles is indicated at the end of the chapter. To achieve principle 6 you need to have knowledge of support networks. The EPP could be one support system, but you also need to know about self-help groups.

Self-help groups

Self-help groups include a wide range of different groups that may be entirely run by patients or may have considerable input from health professionals. The Department of Health also advocated that healthcare professionals should *ensure support is available from a knowledgeable patient as well as broader peer networks and community support* (2005c, p30). This is because it is of great help for patients to talk to someone with experience of being in the same position. A survey by the DH (2005b) found that two-thirds of the people asked said that assistance from people with the same health problem would help them to self-care. However, the same survey found that public generally did not know much about such self-help groups.

Activity 7.5   *Reflection*

Imagine you have a long-term health problem (choose one from your field of nursing).

- What do you think you would gain from accessing a self-help group?
- Do you see any disadvantages in contacting such a group?

Outline answers are given at the end of the chapter.

Activity 7.5 should help you to see the advantages and disadvantages of such groups. Some of these may be dependent on the quality of the group and, in particular, on the facilitators. As well as providing advice, self-help and service provision, the function of some groups is also campaigning and lobbying, and fundraising for research (Coulter, 2002). A recent example of campaigning is the lobbying of NICE by the Alzheimer's Society for drug therapy to be prescribed for early sufferers of dementia, not just those moderately and severely affected. Fundraising for research into their health problem may help people to think that they are doing something positive about their situation. Whether people find these groups useful is an individual choice, but patients and carers can only make that choice if they know about them.

Activity 7.6   *Evidence-based practice and research*

Go to **www.bma.org.uk/patients_public/selfhelporg.jsp**.

Through this BMA site, access the NHS Equip Gateway or National Voices Directory and find a self-help group for a person you have recently nursed. There are also contact details for carer groups.

This is for individual study and no outline answer is provided.

From undertaking Activity 7.6, you should have found just how many groups are available. This number in itself could be said to demonstrate the need for such groups. Some professionals might see this as a criticism of their professional expertise, but you need to remember that they offer a different kind of support that no professional can unless they have experienced the particular condition. If you are truly working with people as partners, you should tell them about all their options so that they can make an informed choice.

People who participate in self-help groups appreciated the sharing of information, experiences and practical solutions (Coulter and Ellins, 2006), even though there is no strong evidence for health improvement from participation in such groups. Carers say they find that membership increases their confidence and ability to cope. They also say that it helps family functioning and makes the burden of care feel lighter. In another study (Arksey, 2003), carers reported high satisfaction with mutual support and activity groups. Sharing experiences helped them to cope and made their outlook more positive. Some self-help groups are large and nationally established, while others are smaller and local (see Chapter 4). An example of such a group is given in the following case study.

Case study

*Beeston Action for Families was set up eight years ago. This is a small, local group of carers and their families that developed out of a social group for people with learning disabilities. Their carers realised that they had shared issues and experiences, which made them decide to set up the group. They have been supported in starting up their group by Health for All. Although they are a small group, they have a wide range of activities, such as going on residential courses and day trips. Their website also shows their increasing involvement with other projects. For more information, go to **www.beestonactionforfamilies.org.uk**.*

Self-help groups support carers to make positive changes in their lives, which enables them to carry on caring. These groups can offer them and people with long-term conditions ways of coping with life. To consolidate what you have learnt in this chapter, try Activity 7.7.

Think of a patient or a carer whom you have recently encountered and who was being supported in order to self-care.

- What support were they given?
- At what time was this offered?
- What forms did this support take?
- Were they given information about self-help groups?
- Find out if there is an information centre or disabled living centre in your area.

This is for individual reflection and no outline answer is provided.

Personalised care planning

Personalised care planning can also promote self-management of long-term health problems. *High Quality Care for All* (Darzi, 2008) announced the intention that *all 15 million people with one or more long-term conditions should be offered a personalised care plan, developed, agreed and regularly reviewed with a lead professional* (p41). These plans are designed to provide personalised and integrated care planning that meets their range of needs. Community matrons provide this fixed point of contact for the patient and have a primary role in working with patients to assess and support their care needs.

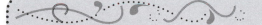

Chapter summary

This chapter has discussed how you promote self-care and self-management for patients and carers. In partnering patients, you need to support them in accessing self-management programmes and self-help resources. Another crucial aspect of supporting self-care and self-management is information-giving. This aspect of partnership working, and health literacy, will be discussed in the next chapter.

Activities: brief outline answers

Activity 7.1 Self-care activities (pages 113–14)

- Activities performed could include washing, dressing, cleaning teeth, brushing hair, going to the toilet, eating, drinking. Did you include any health-enhancing activities such as exercising?
- You probably did not need anyone to help you, but you may have used equipment, e.g. a toothbrush.
- A parent could demonstrate how they performed some of these activities for their child, but may also have talked their child through doing them for themselves, e.g. putting shoes on.
- An older person or disabled person may have needed a carer, which may have reduced their control over such activities.

Activity 7.2 Self-care needs (page 116)

A patient would need (adapted from Murray, 2009, p225):

*   information – what to do, why do it, when to do it;
*   emotional support;
*   social support;
*   behaviour change support – how to do it;
*   decision support – which treatment, what options;
*   monitoring and feedback.

A nurse would need:

*   communication skills;
*   teaching skills;
*   knowledge.

Activity 7.3 Expert Patients Programme (page 117)

*   Possible feelings could include: being unsure, worried about being part of a group of strangers, or nervous about what is involved; wondering if it will help; feeling it is a last resort; being excited by a new opportunity.
*   You would hope to gain more knowledge about health, new skills, more self-confidence and reduced symptoms, e.g. pain, fatigue, anxiety; improved communication with healthcare professionals and more effectiveness in accessing appropriate health and social care services.

It is important that expectations are realistic: it does not offer a cure.

Activity 7.4 Finding out about 'expert patients' (page 119)

If you do not know about what is available in your area, you can visit **www.expertpatients.co.uk/ publications** and find leaflets and posters for informing patients and carers. These include phone enquiry lines to find out about local provision.

Activity 7.5 Self-help groups (page 121)

*   The Department of Health (2008a) states that a self-help group boosts self-confidence, offers practical and emotional support, and encourages you to learn about your condition and think about what might help. You may feel that you are doing something positive, are being active, are helping others, and want to be more self-reliant. You will find out that you are not alone and have an opportunity to identify with other people's experiences. Participation in fund-raising activity may raise your morale.
*   The group may not function well, may wallow in self-pity, and some members may dominate and offer a one-sided perspective. You may not wish to associate with people with the same problem. There may be some mortality of membership.

Further reading

Coulter, A and Ellins, J (2006) Improving self care, in Coulter, A and Ellins, J, *Patient-focused Interventions: A review of the evidence*. London: Health Foundation.

This provides a comprehensive overview of the evidence base for self-care for you to appraise.

Department of Health (DH) (2005) *Supporting Self Care – A Practical Option: Diagnostic, monitoring and assistive devices, technologies and equipment to support self care*. London: DH.

This is a summary of a Review Report and is available online at **www.dh.gov.uk/selfcare**.

Department of Health (DH) (2008) *Raising the Profile of Long Term Conditions Care: A compendium of information*. London: DH.

This is a comprehensive document that focuses on what people with long-term conditions said they wanted from services and giving examples of delivering high-quality personalised care. It is available online at **www.dh.gov.uk/en/Publicationsandstatistics/Publications/PublicationsPolicyAndGuidance/DH_082069**.

EPPCIC (2007) *Self-Management of Long-term Conditions: A handbook for people with chronic disease* (2nd edition). Boulder, CO: Bull Publishing.

The first chapter is about actively self-managing and the second chapter is about resources. The remainder of the book has a range of topics of interest for people who are self-managing long-term conditions.

Skills for Care and Skills for Health (2008) *Common Core Principles to Support Self Care*. Leeds: Skills for Care and Skills for Health.

This is also available at **www.dh.gov.uk** or **www.skillsforcare.org.uk** or **www.skillsforhealth.org.uk**. For each principle, they detail what behaviours are required.

Useful websites

http://patienteducation.stanford.edu/programs/cdsmp.html

This site has further details of Lorig's work at Stanford.

www.dh.gov.uk/SelfCare

This site has more information about the government vision for self-care, initiatives in this field and the range of services available.

www.dh.gov.uk/yourhealth

Access this site for further information about 'Your health, your way', which is designed to help healthcare professionals support patients to self-care.

www.expertpatients.co.uk

This site has further information about the Expert Patients Programme.

www.healthtalkonline.org

This offers patient information, patient stories and patient blogs.

www.patients-association.org.uk

The Patients Association is a national charity. It offers help and advice with online forums for patients to discuss issues and exchange ideas. Sharing ideas may enable people to find solutions to their problems.

www.skillsforcare.org.uk

Download (free) a self-care training pack to help you understand the common core principles for self-care.

www.staying-positive.co.uk

This EPPCIC website is for young people aged 12–18 and provides information on their workshops. These include subjects such as relationships, keeping up with school work, medication and social life. These workshops are designed to help young people meet new friends and get support from others in the same position. It is also to engender confidence in dealing with friends, family and professionals and coping with health services. You can download a DVD about the project.

Chapter 8
Health information and health literacy

NMC Standards for Pre-registration Nursing Education

This chapter will address the following competencies:

Domain 1: Professional values

3. All nurses must support and promote the health, wellbeing, rights and dignity of people, groups, communities and populations. These include people whose lives are affected by ill health, disability, ageing, death and dying. Nurses must understand how these activities influence public health.

6. All nurses must understand the roles and responsibilities of other health and social care professionals and seek to work with them collaboratively for the benefit of all who need care.

Domain 2: Communication and interpersonal skills

2. All nurses must use a range of communication skills and technologies to support person-centred care and enhance quality and safety. They must ensure people receive all the information they need in a language and manner that allows them to make informed choices and share decision making. They must recognise when language interpretation or other communication support is needed and know how to obtain it.

Domain 3: Nursing practice and decision-making

5. All nurses must understand public health principles, priorities and practice in order to recognise and respond to major causes and social determinants of health, illness and health inequalities. They must use a range of information and data to assess the needs of people, groups, communities and populations, and work to improve health, wellbeing and experiences of healthcare; secure equal access to health screening, health promotion and healthcare; and promote social inclusion.

NMC Essential Skills Clusters

This chapter will address the following ESCs:

Cluster: Care, compassion and communication

2. People can trust the newly qualified graduate nurse to engage in person centred care, empowering people to make choices about how their needs are met when they are unable to meet them for themselves.

continued opposite . . .

continued . . .

By the second progression point:

2. Actively empowers people to be involved in the assessment and care planning process.

By entry to the register:

14. Actively helps people to identify and use their strengths to achieve their goals and aspirations.

6. People can trust the newly registered graduate nurse to engage therapeutically and actively listen to their needs and concerns, responding using skills that are helpful, providing information that is clear, accurate, meaningful and free from jargon.

By the first progression point:

1. Communicates effectively both orally and in writing, so that the meaning is always clear.

By entry to the register:

11. Is proactive and creative in enhancing communication and understanding.

8. People can trust the newly registered nurse to gain their consent based on sound understanding and informed choice prior to any intervention and that their rights in decision making and consent will be respected and upheld.

By the second progression point:

3. Ensures that the meaning of consent to treatment and care is understood by the people or service users.

By entry to the register:

4. Uses helpful and therapeutic strategies to enable people to understand treatments and other interventions in order to give informed consent.
6. Assesses and responds to the needs and wishes of carers and relatives in relation to information and consent.

Cluster: Medicines management

35. People can trust the newly registered graduate nurse to work as part of a team to offer holistic care and a range of treatment options of which medicines may form a part.

By entry to the register:

3. Works confidently as part of the team and, where relevant, as leader of the team, to develop treatment options and choices with the person receiving care and their carers.

Chapter aims

By the end of this chapter, you should be able to:

* discuss the role of health information in promoting patient and carer partnership;
* identify sources of health information for patients and carers;

- articulate good practice in producing health information;
- consider ways of evaluating the quality of health information;
- define health literacy;
- debate how health literacy promotes patient and carer partnership.

Introduction

In the last chapter we saw that access to health information is an essential element of self-care and self-management.. Without information, patients and carers cannot make choices. The Department of Health (2004a) stated that high-quality information empowered people and, as a nurse, that is what you will be doing. Therefore, in this chapter we will look at health information, ways in which such information can be transmitted and means of making it easily available. Your role in providing information about medicines will also be discussed. The chapter will also address health literacy and information prescriptions to show how your understanding of these will enhance patient and carer partnership.

When patients have access to both generalised information about health, and personalised information about their specific condition, they are better equipped to improve their health and quality of life and, more importantly, they can *act as equal partners in their care wherever possible* (DH, 2004a, p4). The government again made this commitment to the provision of health information for shared decision-making in *Equity and Excellence* (DH, 2010b) in an NHS information revolution. The aim of this revolution is to provide patients with access to *comprehensive, trustworthy and easy to understand information* (p13). Patients become less empowered when they lack the information they need to make informed decisions (Paterson, 2002).

Why patients want information

Research into the issue of why patients want information found the following reasons.

- *They want explanations of what is wrong.*
- *They need to gain a realistic idea of prognosis.*
- *They want to make the most of consultations.*
- *They want to understand the processes and likely outcomes of possible tests and treatments.*
- *Information can assist them in self-care.*
- *They need to learn about services and sources of help.*
- *Information can provide reassurance and help them to cope.*
- *Information can help others understand.*
- *They need to legitimise their help-seeking and concerns.*
- *Information can identify further infrastructure and self-help groups.*
- *They need to identify the 'best' healthcare providers.*

(Coulter et al., 1998, pp29–30)

This last reason is very much at the forefront of current government policy in providing choice of service. High-quality information is important for all these reasons, and also because it helps people to make an informed choice. Providing high-quality patient information is a priority in the move towards patient involvement in shared decision-making (Entwistle et al., 1997). The results of NHS surveys (Garratt, 2009) showed that 79 per cent of patients reported satisfaction with the amount of information received, but this still means that one in five patients are not satisfied with this. Some of the above reasons are about decision-making and you can think about this in Activity 8.1.

Activity 8.1   *Decision-making*

- What constitutes an informed choice?
- What influences are there on making an informed choice?

Outline answers are given at the end of the chapter.

Activity 8.1 was designed to help you explore the relationship between information and patient choice. Informed consent, a concept that you will have discussed in the ethical content of your course, is closely related to this and is also dependent on the quality of information provided.

Access to health information

Before discussing the production of health information, you need to think about its accessibility. Although there is plenty of information, patients and carers are often given no guidance on how to find it (Picker Institute, 2007). In particular, healthcare professionals can be poor at helping patients find voluntary area support groups and information about support for family and carers. You will remember from the last chapter the importance of self-help groups. People need to know about them; it is reported that nearly all patients want information about family relationships, but more than half of them say that this is not given (McCaughan and Thompson, 2000). This is particularly significant for day case patients, as it is the relatives who are central to their care.

All this means that you need to think not only about the health information itself, but also how you help people gain access to it. Patients and carers value staff who provide access to information about day-to-day issues (Wollin et al., 2006).

Activity 8.2 is designed to start you thinking about this.

Activity 8.2   *Communication*

Suppose you had a health problem and wanted information about it.

• Where would you go to find this?
• In what form would you want this information?
• What qualities would you look for in this information?

Outline answers are given at the end of the chapter.

In carrying out Activity 8.2, you will have thought about your own personal preferences, but your patients and their carers may have others. You may have chosen IT access, but remember that the greatest users of health services are the elderly and this may not be an option for them. Access to health information is the foundation on which patients and carers can be actively involved in their care (Coulter and Ellins, 2006). The Department of Health (2004a) stated that there was a need for healthcare professionals to be more proactive in their approach to making health information available to patients and carers. Also, there are half a million people in the UK for whom English is not a first language, and you need to consider their access too; you should find out about local translation and interpretation services. So accessibility is also about the form in which information is presented, which should include Braille and audio for the visually impaired.

Internet sources

The Department of Health (2004a) makes improving access to information a priority. Included within this is the issue of patients having access to their own health records. In their strategy (2004a, p10) they identify the following ways of increasing this access:

• NHS Direct Interactive;
• Health Direct;
• Health search engine;
• nationally procured information resources;
• information to help choose a hospital for elective care.

How much do you know about the first three of these? If you are unsure, look these up in *Better Information, Better Choices, Better Health* (2004a), which is accessible on **www.dh.gov.uk**. The nationally procured information services were designed to enable patients and carers to have access to the same evidence-based materials as professionals. They are also designed to help healthcare professionals to provide up-to-date and consistent information and treatment options to patients. Since then, the government has developed digital access, such as NHS Choices, which is *a shop window, providing the opportunity to inform and engage patients, people who use services, carers and the public* (DH, 2008c, p13). We will return to these later in the chapter when looking at information prescriptions.

Some of these government initiatives rely on the internet, which of course can convey huge amounts of information. Patients and carers use the internet for emotional and social support, for example from online blogs on social networking sites such as Facebook, Bebo and mySpace. Cancerbackup has developed a site for teenagers at **www.click4tic.org.uk**, which allows users to set up their own page. As well as communicating with other teenagers, they can ask a nurse questions.

Case study

Mandy was 24 when she was diagnosed with acute lymphoblastic leukaemia. She and her family were devastated at her diagnosis. She imagined that she was the only girl her age with cancer, but when she used sites such as the ones described she found that there were others living with this too, and she was helped by tips as to how to cope with problems such as hair loss.

Just as texting was found useful by the specialist nurse in Chapter 3, use of these sites can be very beneficial as the case study illustrates. More interactive uses of the internet include accessing self-assessment tools with feedback, online consultations and internet interventions. These will be discussed again later in the chapter when the subject of information prescriptions is addressed. There are 15.4 million people in the UK with a long-term condition (DH, 2005c), but many of these are elderly and may not have access to the internet. So, while it is a useful resource, you must be careful not to just glibly refer patients and carers to websites. Sites also vary in quality (DH, 2004a; Edwards et al., 2009), so encourage patients and carers to think carefully about which sites they visit, and to concentrate on recognised, organised and impartial organisations. Further information about this is available at the end of the chapter.

Verbal sources

You may have wanted to talk about your problem with a healthcare professional. Written information should never replace this form of communication, but is useful in backing up what has been said. To assess your skills in giving verbal information, try Activity 8.3.

Activity 8.3   *Communication*

Find a friend to help you with this. You will need to give him or her a piece of paper and a pen. Sit comfortably back to back or in such a way that your friend cannot see the following diagram.

Ask your friend to draw the object on a sheet of paper as you describe it. When he or she has finished, compare this with the original.

- Identify what issues there are for information-giving.

An outline answer is given at the end of the chapter.

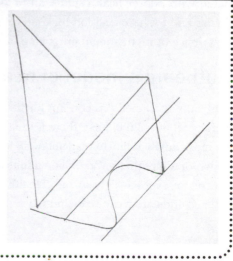

One of the difficulties you may have identified in Activity 8.3 is that this object was not recognisable to either of you. Therefore, you could not start by saying, for example, 'I want you to draw me a house.' If you could have started with this common understanding, the task would have been easier. In healthcare, however, you often have to give patients and carers information about subjects they have never heard of before. This should help you to realise how important it is to assess what they need to know or what they already know about the subject first, so that you can start at their level. You then need to plan how to deliver the information. Organise it logically; think about what equipment they may need before telling them what they need to do with it. Then, as you explain, ensure that they understand by asking them to repeat, in their own words, what you have said. Activity 8.3 demonstrates the importance of understanding what is said.

Patients and carers also need to be able to utilise written information where similar issues arise. Therefore, we need to consider health literacy.

What is health literacy?

Health literacy is a key component of the government's strategy for improving the nation's health. The aim of building strong partnerships in care can only be achieved through greater health literacy (Darzi, 2008); but what do we mean by health literacy? At first, this term appears simple: if literacy is about the ability to read and write, you just add health and then it means the ability to read and write about health; but over the past 20 years, the concept had been widened (Gray, 2009). More than just the ability to read health pamphlets, it is the *cognitive and social skills which determine the motivation and ability of individuals to gain access to, understand and use information in ways which promote and maintain good health* (Nutbeam, 1998, p357).

Health literacy is central for patients who want to self-care, because they need to obtain, process and understand health information (Coulter and Ellins, 2006). Health literacy fosters patient participation and empowerment (Nutbeam, 1998), while low levels of health literacy are associated with poorer health status, and reduced ability to communicate with healthcare professionals and to share decision-making (Coulter and Ellins (2006). People with low health literacy experience more treatment errors and take more medication.

Nutbeam's model of health literacy

Nutbeam developed this concept further when he went on to describe differing levels of health literacy (2000, p263). First, there is the level described as *functional health literacy*, which concerns the individual's ability to read and write in order to function in the healthcare setting. You should remember here that seven million adults in this country have literacy and numeracy skills below that of an average 11 year old (Health Link, 2004, cited in DH, 2004a). Never assume that patients and carers can read and write, as indicated in this case study.

> ## Case study
>
> *Mary Brown was newly diagnosed with Type 2 diabetes. The practice nurse at the GP clinic educated her in how to manage her condition and gave her literature to read to support what she told her about testing her blood glucose levels. But, as the weeks went by, Mary appeared to make little progress. Then, after several months, Mary's daughter had a quiet word with the nurse to explain that her mother could not read or write.*

In your nursing practice you need to be aware of patients' level of literacy, but you also need to be aware that functional health literacy is not just a translation of basic literacy skills into a health setting. Such skills do contribute, but health literacy is context-specific. This means, for example, that people with high-level literacy skills such as graduates, but who are not familiar with healthcare, may not benefit from the same level of health literacy skills because of unfamiliar language, jargon or anxiety.

To return to Nutbeam's model (2000), his second level is *interactive health literacy*. This requires more advanced literacy and social skills to be able to actively participate in healthcare. This then requires a model of education where people are actively engaged rather than being passive. Finally, he describes *critical health literacy*, where people are able critically to analyse and use information to overcome structural barriers to health.

So, how is the health literacy of the nation? Research in 2007 by von Wagner et al. (2007) used **TOFHLA** (Test of Functional Health Literacy in Adults) and found that 11.4 per cent of their study participants had either marginal or inadequate functional health literacy. Limitations in health literacy increased with age, low educational status and low income. Therefore, you need to be particularly aware of the vulnerability of these groups in not being able to access and utilise health information.

Health information

Adult literacy campaigns have been operating in the UK for over 30 years to help improve generic literacy, which should impact on health literacy; there are also TV campaigns on health literacy. These are beyond the scope of this book, but, as a health professional, you need to be aware of them. The concept of health literacy is also associated with self-management, which was discussed in the last chapter. The high-level skill of being able to appraise health information and apply it in your own context is called critical health literacy, and it is perhaps unrealistic to expect patients and carers to achieve this level of skill (Edwards et al., 2009). Instead, patients need high-quality information; to improve health literacy, *high quality health information materials need to be accessible, readable and comprehensible for the general public* (Edwards et al., 2009, p102). So, while improving health literacy is about more than just giving information, information was still the foundation (Nutbeam, 2000). Therefore, we now focus on health information and different ways of presenting information resources. To do this, it may be useful to draw on your own experience in Activity 8.4.

Activity 8.4   *Critical thinking*

Find a health information pamphlet about a subject that you are not familiar with.

- What is good about the way information is given?
- What features could be improved?

Outline answers are given at the end of the chapter.

Activity 8.4 was designed to encourage you to think about information from a patient's or carer's perspective. A patient needs information that is different from the kind a professional needs (Entwistle et al., 1997) and so it is helpful if patients are involved throughout the process of information production (Coulter et al., 1998). Focus groups are a good means of identifying the information needs of patients and carers, and then they can help with design and content. Design may have influenced which leaflet you selected for the activity. You need to think about how patient information is designed not only so that you can ensure the leaflets you use with patients are of high quality, but also because, when you qualify, you may be involved in designing leaflets or posters for your area of practice. Here is a set of questions you should ask yourself before launching into this task.

- *WHY are you proposing to develop information materials? What do you intend to achieve by them?*
- *WHO are the intended recipients of the information?*
- *WHAT information do you intend to provide? Have you any evidence that the intended recipients would find it useful?*
- *HOW will you present the information? What media will you use, what language, etc.?*
- *WHEN, WHERE, HOW and BY WHOM will the information be given?*
- *How will you ensure the QUALITY of the information package you produce?*
    (Entwistle et al., 1997, p71)

This is a useful outline of the whole process of information production. The first point is asking you to think clearly about the purpose of your information and whether it already exists or not. Considering your target audience is essential in starting you thinking about their requirements and making sure that what you do is pertinent to their needs. This is closely followed by the question of ensuring that these *are* their needs by asking them, as previously discussed. You also need to be sensitive to religious, cultural, ethical and gender issues. Communication needs to reflect the characteristics of the target audience. The next two questions relate to production issues, which we will discuss in more detail. The last question, about evaluation and quality issues, will be addressed in the next chapter.

Designing health information

In the questions above, you are asked to think about the most appropriate media to use. If you were working with children or people with learning difficulties, you would use more pictures, or maybe a DVD or video. Further information on working with these groups can be found at the end of the chapter. Returning to our discussion of literacy levels, your choice of language needs to be careful and you must avoid jargon, which creeps in so easily (which was identified as a problem for patient involvement in Chapter 3). Do you recall the handover on your first practice learning shift? Was it full of unintelligible terminology, which in a short time became quite familiar? Even simple words like 'pyrexia' are unknown to most patients and carers. This is why it is important to involve patients and carers in the production of information. Make it user-friendly by using 'you', 'we', etc. and everyday language. Make it interactive by using realistic dialogue, or a question and answer format. Check that your tone is not authoritarian ('you must stick to this diet'), victim blaming ('you will only have yourself to blame if you do not do this') or scaremongering ('forgetting a tablet will have serious consequences').

You can assess your draft writing with a readability scoring system, which is a formula that calculates the complexity of language. One example would be the Flesch Reading Ease score, which is a measurement based on the number of words in a sentence and the number of syllables per 100 words (Mumford, 1997). Mumford went on to identify that, while these scores were useful in identifying the reading grade of a piece of literature, they do not, of course, help in knowing the reading age of the patient. They are also mechanistic and do not help with identifying the clarity of meaning. Think about the patient's or carer's journey and make the order of your material logical in its development. Content should flow and have meaning.

In order to help professionals to produce high-quality information, the Department of Health produced a Toolkit (DH, 2003b). To explore this Toolkit, you should try Activity 8.5.

Activity 8.5   *Communication*

- Select a topic relevant to a patient or carer in your clinical practice.
- Access the DH Toolkit at **www.dh.gov.uk/en/Publicationsandstatistics/ Publications/PublicationsPolicyAndGuidance/DH_4070141** and note its recommendations.
- Design a leaflet to provide information about this topic.
- Are there any other alternative formats you could have used?

Some suggestions are given at the end of the chapter.

Activity 8.5 shows you just how many things there are to think about in producing high-quality patient information. Did you think about making your leaflet pertinent to your local area? Did you indicate further sources of support for the reader? There should also be local contact details. Did you leave a space for people to note their own questions for their next meeting with a health professional?

Further suggestions for resources to help in producing health information are given at the end of the chapter. In order to ensure that they include the right information, researchers have involved patients and carers in the production and evaluation process.

Research summary: Patient DVD on Understanding Angioplasty

This joint research project by the University of Leeds and clinical staff from Leeds THT aimed to gather data in order to provide angioplasty patients and their families with a patient-centred information resource. The DVD would take viewers through the 'patient journey', with explanations and commentary from patients, carers and healthcare professionals about what to expect when being treated with planned coronary angioplasty. The DVD was also to help patients make important lifestyle changes.

Aims: to explore the way in which people self-manage their lifestyle after coronary angioplasty. Emphasis was given to understanding the complexity of factors that patients' self-management of lifestyle factors identified.

Methods: a series of one-to-one interviews with 26 participants recruited from a specialist cardiac centre after coronary angioplasty. Each participant was interviewed in a home setting at 1–2 weeks and 6–8 weeks after hospital discharge. The average age of participants was 61.8 years (range 48–85); 55 per cent were male. Interviews were audio-taped and transcribed verbatim. NVivo software was used to systematically order and synthesise findings.

Results: Participants generally attributed coronary heart disease to lifestyle factors. However, the way in which they interpreted this information within their own personal context varied, and did not consistently reflect their individual coronary risk factor profile. Coronary angioplasty was seen as an effective 'repair' for clogged arteries. Participants generally recognised the benefits of lifestyle changes, but were less clear about how such changes could be achieved. Few had the skills to set and review lifestyle change goals. They lacked detailed information about dietary change and how far they could 'push' with physical activity levels. They were often uncertain about when hospital care ended and whether other support was available. Co-existing conditions such as diabetes and obesity made dietary change and physical activity a challenge.

We used the findings from the above study, combined with existing clinical guidelines, to develop a patient-centred DVD.

(Project Lead: Dr Felicity Astin, School of Healthcare, University of Leeds)

From this, you can see the importance of interdisciplinary working. You should also think about contacting other Trusts to see whether work can be shared and that you are not reinventing the wheel.

Asking questions

Have you ever been in a healthcare situation where, the minute you left, you remembered an important question you had wanted to ask? One way in which you can encourage patients to be involved in decision-making is to encourage them to prepare questions about their care in advance, as often, when their appointment comes, they may forget what they were going to ask. The Department of Health (2004a) reported that 43 per cent of patients never wrote questions down prior to an appointment. They identified that one way to empower people was to help them make the most of their appointments by offering *an essential set of questions to ask* (p17). When you are in practice, encourage patients to use these and to think about which are the most important to them. You can access a useful list of possible questions at NHS Choices (**www.nhs. uk/nhsengland/aboutnhsservices/questionstoask/pages/makethemostofyour appointment.aspx**). If patients or carers do not have internet access, design a sheet based on these questions for distribution to them. Within *Better Information, Better Choices, Better Health* (DH, 2004a) there was also a commitment to establish information prescriptions.

Information prescriptions

Following its commitment to these in *Our Health, Our Care, Our Say* (DH, 2006a), there were pilot schemes set up to deliver information prescriptions to people with long-term conditions. The DH set out five key components of the process, which were:

- the content should come from relevant and reliable sources;
- they would be personalised to the individual;
- links could be created to other directories of information;
- they would be dispensed by health professionals;
- they would be accessible via a range of channels.

There has been ongoing evaluation from the pilot schemes, but it is the intention that, eventually, these prescriptions will be available to everyone with a long-term condition. Ask about these when you are in clinical practice.

NHS Choices

NHS Choices is a source of personalised digital services designed to improve patient and carer services so as to enable people to access appropriate information about their health and social needs. To find out more about these services, try Activity 8.6.

Activity 8.6   *Communication*

- Visit **www.nhs.uk/choices** and see the wide range of services offered.
- Now go to **www.nhs.uk/Planners/Yourhealth/Pages/Information.aspx** and click on the link to create a prescription yourself.

This is for individual study and no outline answer is provided.

In undertaking Activity 8.6, you can see how information-giving has developed to embrace systems that people use in their everyday lives. Patients are encouraged by NHS Choices to communicate with healthcare professionals via text, YouTube, etc. (DH, 2008c) and it suggests that the healthcare professional could download a relevant page or prescription for patients without internet access. It reports how patients are enabled to self-care by having online monitoring services for conditions such as asthma – they can share their results and have a review with the asthma nurse online. This should help more patients to access expert advice and support. When you are in clinical practice, especially in the community, find out what services are being offered, and how patients and carers are informed of these. Following test results and monitoring, patients and carers may need advice about their medication and this is what we will discuss next.

Information about medicines

The Department of Health (2005c) identified patient advice about medicines as being important in self-management, and found that only half of patients with long-term conditions took their medicines as prescribed. Nurses are good at providing information on medication (Martens, 1998), but although giving medication accounts for 9.3 per cent of nurses' total working time (Whittington and McLaughlin, 2000), this time is spent in physical administration and recording, rather than interacting with patients about these medicines. You need to think about this usage of time to ensure maximum benefit for patients. If you are waiting while a patient takes medication, you could use this time to explore what they think about it. If people have misgivings about their medication, or misunderstandings about its purpose, this can affect how they take it. You could also check their knowledge of their medication. Talking to patients in this way is an example of what the NMC (2008b) means when it states that the administration of medicines is not a simply a mechanistic task.

There has also been research on what kind of information people want about their medicine; Martens (1998) found that people wanted written and oral information. Written information should not replace verbal consultation (Grime et al., 2007), but this information should be individualised. People wanted the information about the medication contextualised to their illness; Martens recommended that the information should be based on *patient assessment of their knowledge, learning ability, what he or she wants to know and the specifications and risks of prescribed medication* (1998, p347). Knowledge could be assessed by asking them what they know, for example 'Tell me about your tablets.' You can assess a patient's learning ability by noting their concentration levels, use of language and what they read. Use open questions to find out what they want to know. You need to think about making the specifications of the medication personal by relating these to their daily routine, for example when they get up, and, finally, explaining what to look out for in terms of side effects. As you can see, there is a lot to cover, which is why you need to give the information over time, and repeat it, and check that the patient or carer has understood. Personalised medication charts and colour coding of medicines can help to reinforce this (Martens, 1998).

Patients who do not take their medicines as prescribed have sometimes been described as 'noncompliant', but this term has connotations of the passive patient not having followed a healthcare professional's instructions. 'Concordance' is a better word, as this suggests a *collaborative process of decision-making regarding treatment* (Gray and Robson, 2002, p1). But this is more than just terminology; it is about how you treat people and whether you just expect people to follow your expert advice or whether you act in a way that engages people in the process that will enhance their understanding. When you take a patient-focused approach you need to identify patient information needs and this will improve concordance (Shuttleworth, 2004). Nurses need to listen to patients and understand their view of the medication. Failing to discuss medication fully with patients, and not checking that they understand, can give rise to risky situations, as described in the following case study.

Case study

During his stay for treatment of a deep vein thrombosis, John was stabilised on an anti-coagulant. Shortly after his discharge, he was readmitted and his clotting times were found to be very high, putting him in great danger of bleeding. When asked about how he had taken his medication, he explained that, on discharge, the nurse had told him that 'These tablets are for the pain in your leg.' As his pain had returned, he had taken some tablets and, when this did not take his pain away, he took some more . . ..

You can see how important it is to explain clearly to the patient the relationship between their condition and the medication. John thought that, if the tablets were for his pain, he could take them like painkillers, which could have had disastrous consequences. Garratt (2009) found that only 30 per cent of patients had been informed of side effects to watch out for on discharge.

While written information is designed by drug companies and pharmacists, you need to think about how you inform patients about their medication. Think about this in Activity 8.7.

Activity 8.7   *Communication*

Imagine that you are a 50-year-old man who is hypertensive. You have been prescribed a beta-blocker for hypertension.

- What information would you want about this medication?
- How should this information be given?
- Do you read the information in any medication you take?
- What might influence whether you took your medication as prescribed?

Outline answers are given at the end of the chapter.

Activity 8.7 was designed to enable you to use your own experience to appreciate your role in medication administration. Here, how the information is presented will mirror the healthcare professional's perspective on administration. In their review of the literature, Grime et al. (2007) found that some professionals took a patient education approach with the intention of increasing compliance, while others saw their role as engaging with patients to empower them to make their own decisions about medicines. They also found that patients did not always ask questions. Therefore, you need to encourage patients to think about what they want to know about their medication, and encourage them to write this down so that they remember to ask their doctor or pharmacist.

Activity 8.8   *Reflection*

- On your practice learning opportunities, who discusses medication with patients and carers?
- How is this done and for how long?
- Are patients encouraged to be involved in the medication-giving process while in hospital?

Outline answers are given at the end of the chapter.

This activity was designed to help you to realise the importance of interprofessional working and how essential this is to medication information. People need time to digest the information and to think what questions to ask. Do not hurry them, but deliver the information over a period of time. Also, always consider the carer role and their need for information. Although you are not designing the medicine information, you should be ensuring that patients and carers have the information they want and supporting them to ask appropriate questions of a relevant practitioner if they need to. You want them to have good-quality information, and so we next think about measures of quality.

The information standard

As suggested earlier in the chapter, it is not easy for people to reach a level of critical health literacy. To help people identify reliable and trustworthy information, the government has developed an information standard mark scheme, open to health and social care information producers. Participation in the scheme is voluntary across the public, non-for-profit and commercial sectors. Organisations that meet the criteria of this mark will be able to use it on their materials. The scheme is focused on people in England but, because many organisations offer literature across all countries in the UK, and because this standard can also apply to websites, this information will be more widely available. You can find more information on this standard on the website indicated at the end of the chapter. Also, you need to think about developing your own appraisal skills so that you can advise patients and carers about the quality of information.

Activity 8.9 is designed to help you relate what the chapter has discussed to your clinical practice.

Activity 8.9   *Critical thinking*

- While respecting confidentiality, identify a patient with a long-term health problem in your clinical area.
- Think about what will be their future, ongoing needs ensuing from this health problem.
- Identify services available to them, e.g. voluntary, social, charitable, LA, self-help, NHS.
- Appraise the relevant information that there is in the clinical area and how this was used with them.

This is for individual reflection and no outline answer is provided.

> ## Chapter summary
>
> This chapter has discussed how health literacy can improve patient and carer involvement in their care and promote self-care. It has encouraged you to consider how health information is produced and utilised to facilitate shared decision-making. While there has been some discussion of the quality of the information, these issues will be addressed in the next chapter.

Activities: brief outline answers

Activity 8.1 Making informed choices (page 129)

Informed choice means that the decision-maker has relevant information, the choice reflects their values and there is enactment of choice (Edwards and Elwyn, 2009).

Informed choice may not be possible, because of, for example, biased or poor-quality information, cultural and personal values, or education. Or no choice may be given, as in the imposition of water fluoridation.

Activity 8.2 Finding and evaluating information (page 130)

- You could gain information from a healthcare professional, NHS Direct, a supermarket, the internet, the media, other people, self-help groups, for example.
- Information should be available in written, verbal, visual and audio forms.
- Information should be clear, attractive and well constructed.

Activity 8.3 Giving verbal information (page 131)

Issues could include:

- meaning – it is difficult to describe an object without a name;
- care with words used – you both understood 'parallel', for example, but words might not have a common meaning or be understood.
- importance of feedback – it was difficult when you could not see what your friend was doing, but you could ask if he or she understood;
- non-verbal deprivation;
- speed of giving information;
- working out where to start and how to deliver the information – logical sequencing.

Activity 8.4 Evaluating a pamphlet (page 134)

- Good features could include: the style it was written in, the font, clear layout, clarity of language.
- Features needing improvement could include: too much or too little information, no further sources of help offered, difficult to understand.

Activity 8.5 Using the Toolkit to design a leaflet (page 135)

- The Toolkit recommends using short sentences, lower case letters, present and active tenses, question and answer format, bulleted or numbered points, small blocks of text, large bold fond for emphasis, a font size no less than 12 point, and diagrams and pictures.
- Alternative formats include Braille, audio, large print or web-based; would an electronic version be useful?

Activity 8.7 Information about medication (page 139)

- Information should include what is was, why you were taking it, how to take it, for how long and any side effects. Why was it the appropriate medication for your condition?
- The medication should be discussed with a health professional, backed up by a clear leaflet.
- You might be influenced by the credibility of the professional, personal values or your decision with regard to costs versus benefits.

Activity 8.8 Discussing medication (page 140)

- Medication is probably discussed with doctors, pharmacists or nurses.
- Discussions should take place on more than one occasion.
- Patients should at least be involved in the discussion but may self-medicate in some circumstances – see the NMC *Standards for Medicines Management* (2008b).

Further reading

Coulter, A and Ellins, J (2006) *Patient Focused Interventions: A review of the evidence.* London: The Health Foundation.

Chapter 2 discusses the evidence base for health literacy.

Coulter, A, Entwistle, V and Gilbert, D (1998) Informing Patients: An assessment of the quality of patient information materials. London: King's Fund.

Chapter 9 contains the main recommendations, Chapter 10 looks at patient evaluation of materials for patients with back pain and Chapter 12 does the same for people with depression.

Hubley, J and Copeman, J (2008) *Practical Health Promotion.* Cambridge: Polity Press.

For further information on promoting health. Chapter 5 is a useful guide to health promotion on a one-to-one basis and Chapter 6 for groups.

Royal College of Nursing (RCN) (2010) *Putting Information at the Heart of Nursing Care: How IT is revolutionising health care.* London: RCN.

Further explanation and information on the use of technology as a medium for providing patient information.

Useful websites

www.evidence.nhs.uk

This offers free access to credible medical sources and the latest health information updates.

www.healthinsite.gov.au

This site contains information about how to assess online health information.

www.leedsanimation.org.uk

This has a range of DVDs for people with learning difficulties. These were made in consultation with Mencap, CHANGE and the NHS.

www.luto.co.uk

This is the website of an organisation established to improve medication information for patients and involves patients in this process. If you are interested in helping to devise patient-friendly medication information or to find out more about efforts to produce this, visit this site.

www.nhsidentity.nhs.uk

This is for further information on producing leaflets. It also includes resources, logos and other materials.

www.pifonline.org.uk

This is the Patient Information Forum site and will give more details on health literacy and medicine information. You can download a *Guide to Appraising Health Information*, which offers tips to help you think about the production of health information. It also contains details of the Information Standard. A search under 'Children' will give ideas of how to make information relevant to this age group.

www.plainenglish.co.uk

The Plain English Campaign provides a free guide on how to write in plain English. It also provides further information on Crystal Mark Standards, which are seals of approval for clarity of documentation.

Chapter 9
Quality issues in patient participation

┌───┐

NMC Standards for Pre-registration Nursing Education

Domain 1: Professional values

7. All nurses must be responsible and accountable for keeping their knowledge and skills up-to-date through continuing professional development. They must aim to improve their performance and enhance the safety and quality of care through evaluation, supervision and appraisal.

Domain 2: Communication and interpersonal skills

7. All nurses must maintain accurate, clear and complete records, including the use of electronic formats, using appropriate and plain language.

Domain 3: Nursing practice and decision-making

1. All nurses must use up-to-date knowledge and evidence to assess, plan, deliver and evaluate care, communicate findings, influence change and promote health and best practice. They must make person-centred, evidence-based judgments and decisions, in partnership with others involved in the care process, to ensure high quality care. They must be able to recognise when the complexity of clinical decisions requires specialist knowledge and expertise, and consult or refer accordingly.

10. All nurses must evaluate their care to improve clinical decision-making, quality and outcomes, using a range of methods, amending the plan of care, where necessary, and communicating changes to others.

Domain 4: Leadership, management and team working

2. All nurses must systematically evaluate care and ensure that they and others use the findings to help improve people's experience and care outcomes and to shape future services.

3. All nurses must be able to identify priorities and manage time and resources effectively to ensure the quality of care is maintained or enhanced.

4. All nurses must be self-aware and recognise how their own values, principles an assumptions may affect their practice. They must maintain their own personal and professional development, learning from experience, through supervision, feedback reflection and evaluation.

└───┘

NMC Essential Skills Clusters

This chapter will address the following ESCs:

Cluster: Care, compassion and communication

5. People can trust the newly registered graduate nurse to engage with them in a warm, sensitive and compassionate way.

By the first progression point:

5. Evaluates ways in which own interactions affect relationships to ensure that they do not impact inappropriately on others.

By entry to the register:

13. Through reflection and evaluation demonstrates commitment to personal and professional life-long learning.

Cluster: Organisational aspects of care

10. People can trust the newly registered graduate nurse to deliver nursing interventions and evaluate their effectiveness against the agreed assessment and care plan.

By the second progression point:

1. Acts collaboratively with people and their carers, enabling and empowering them to take a shared and active role in the delivery and evaluation of nursing interventions.

By entry to the register:

9. Evaluates the effect of interventions, taking account of people's and carers' interpretation of physical, emotional and behavioural changes.

12. People can trust the newly qualified graduate nurse to respond to their feedback and a wide range of sources to learn, develop and improve services.

By the second progression point:

2. Responds appropriately when people want to complain, providing assistance and support.

By entry to the register:

5. Shares complaints, compliments and comments with the team in order to improve care.
6. Actively responds to feedback.
7. Supports people who wish to complain.
8. As an individual team member and team leader, actively seeks and learns from feedback to enhance care and own and others' professional development.
9. Works within ethical and legal frameworks and local policies to deal with complaints, compliments and concerns.

> ## Chapter aims
>
> By the end of this chapter, you should be able to:
>
> * discuss the process of evaluation;
> * debate different approaches to quality measurement;
> * identify policy on quality assurance;
> * discuss patient and carer involvement in quality measurement.

Introduction

This chapter is about evaluating the quality of the work we do as nurses in partnership with patients. First, we will revisit the nursing process and look at the role of evaluation in making sure that we see the patient and carer perspective on the quality of their care. Then we will discuss the concepts of quality and patient satisfaction. Having addressed these, we need to consider how they are measured and how patients and carers should be involved in this process. Various approaches to quality will be outlined and you will be encouraged to examine these in the context of your practice. Finally, we will look at organisations and policy concerned with quality issues.

What is evaluation?

Remember that, in Chapter 1, we discussed the nursing process and evaluation as one of its stages. Evaluation can be seen as *a judgment of the effectiveness of care given against the goals set* (Hogston and Marjoram, 2007, p19), and it is so important that some think there is little point in planning and delivering care if the benefits to the recipient are not examined (Roper et al., 2000); so the evaluation stage is crucial. Evaluation is important because it identifies the value of nursing care (Walsh, 1998). Focusing on quality is an opportunity and a challenge for nurses to identify what we do and demonstrate the outcome of nursing (Beasley, 2010). The nursing process is about more than individualising care – it is also about the professionalisation of nursing and accountability – and evaluation is also concerned with quality assurance (Walsh, 1998). So you can see that, if we are going to look at quality issues in patient and carer involvement, we need to start by thinking about how nursing care is evaluated.

> ## Activity 9.1   *Communication*
>
> * List all the ways you have seen patient care evaluated in your clinical practice.
> * How often was this done?
> * Who was involved in the evaluation?
>
> *Some suggestions are given at the end of the chapter.*

In thinking about what you have seen, you need also to consider the strengths and weaknesses of these practices. There is also the question of when evaluation takes place: the suggested times are at *handover, on reflection, patient satisfaction or complaint and review of the care plan* (Hogston and Marjoram, 2007, p19). The last one is the most popular, and the best plan is to start by looking at goal attainment, and also review your nursing interventions for effectiveness. You might even return to the patient assessment to ensure that it is complete. We will look at patient satisfaction and complaints later in this chapter.

In thinking about nursing handover as an evaluative mechanism, remember what was discussed in Chapter 3 about patient involvement in handover. Patients and families should be involved wherever possible because the problem is theirs, after all (Murray and Atkinson, 2000). If you do not involve people in judgements about their care, you do not have a complete picture.

In thinking about how frequently evaluation takes place, you may have said 'all the time' and, at its best, evaluation is an ongoing process (Llewellyn and Hayes, 2008). Continuous evaluation may be informal, and then formal evaluation is the one that is recorded. Nurses make mental evaluations while they deliver care, and make different recorded evaluations (Walsh, 1998). Mental evaluations could be a reflective activity. Now, reflect on your evaluative skills by considering your strengths and weaknesses.

Activity 9.2   *Reflection*

Reflect on your ability by placing a cross to mark your position on the continuum.

1. How aware am I of identifying emotions or non-verbal behaviour?

    Completely unaware ———————————————————— Totally aware

2. How precise am I in written communication?

    Completely imprecise ——————————————————— Totally precise

3. How effective am I in listening and responding to communication?

    Completely ineffective ——————————————————— Completely effective

4. Do I refer back to care plan goals?

    Never ————————————————————————————— Always

5. Do I talk to patients and carers as part of my evaluation?

    Never ————————————————————————————— Always

6. Do I seek out patients' and carers' views by other means?

    Never ————————————————————————————— Always

7. Do I search out evidence or research when care has not been effective?

    Never ————————————————————————————— Always

8. Do I discuss evaluation findings with patients and their carers?

    Never ————————————————————————————— Always

This is for individual reflection and no outline answer is provided.

As a result of your reflection in Activity 9.2, you may wish to discuss the development of your evaluative skills with your mentor. This is the least popular stage of the nursing process, because you may discover in your evaluation that care has not met the expected standards and this can leave you feeling uncomfortable. Try to realise that this may be due to factors beyond your control and try not to take non-achievement as failure. If you start to feel negatively about evaluation, you may then seek to avoid it, but it is an essential element of nursing. Instead, remember what was discussed about learning with patients and from their experiences, and try to use this constructively to develop your practice. Thinking about the accountability associated with the nursing process should help you to realise that achieving high-quality nursing care is the responsibility of each and every nurse.

Evaluating health information

In the last chapter, we discussed how important it was to develop health information with patients and carers to enable their participation in care. They also need to be involved in evaluating health information.

Activity 9.3   *Communication*

Imagine that you have designed a leaflet about self-care following a tonsillectomy.

- How would you evaluate it?
- What aspects of the leaflet would you consider?

An outline answer is given at the end of the chapter.

Quality

Did you include patient or carer feedback in your evaluation of health information? Evaluating care in the nursing process is at the level of the individual patient and carer, but the overall standard of care needs also to be appraised (Murray and Atkinson, 2000). You may have seen clinical audit and the work of audit teams when you have been in practice. Clinical audit is about reviewing care against agreed standards. These standards could be ones that are nationally agreed, such as the NMC standards, or ones that have been defined at a local level; we will look at an example of these later in the chapter. First, it may be useful to spend a little time thinking about what is meant by 'quality'.

Quality may not be a single attribute but may need to be considered from a range of perspectives (Donabedian, 1980). It has different meanings to different people (Ford and Walsh, 1994); its definition is subjective and influenced by the definer. In other words, what is good quality to one person may be poor to another. It may also be influenced by the context, which is worth considering when you think about when and where you obtain feedback from patients and carers. How honest the feedback is will depend on how free people feel to give it. In healthcare, there could be two different perspectives: from those providing care and from those receiving care.

All too often we measure quality by criteria imposed by the professionals – waiting times, numbers of staff and well-conducted procedures (Hart, 1996), when we should assess quality more from the perspective of the consumer. It has taken a long time for the experiences of patients to be taken into consideration in definitions of quality (Richards and Coulter, 2007). A definition of quality that is now internationally recognised comes from the US Institute of Medicine, and it has six criteria: *patient-centred, safe, effective, timely, efficient and equitable* (Richards and Coulter, 2007, p19). If you accepted this definition you would, of course, then have to think about what patient-centred care means and that could lead to an intense and protracted debate. Patient groups see this to mean services that listen to patients, taking their views seriously, and also attending to the *fundamentals* of care. Richards and Coulter list these fundamentals as *dignity and respect for individuals; well-organised care; clean wards; and nutritious food* (2007, p20). You may remember that the first two of these were discussed as central tenets of care in Chapter 1. It is important to see quality through the eyes of the person receiving care and their families/carers, as illustrated in the following case study.

Case study

John died recently. He died in a pair of hospital pyjamas that did not fit him. They were in a colour he never wore and, although they had been laundered, they were marked with food stains from a previous patient. You might think that this was because John had been admitted as an emergency, or had no pyjamas of his own or no one to bring these in for him, but it wasn't. His daughter had brought several pairs of pyjamas in for him but the nurse who was admitting him had told her to take them home again, saying that 'it was better to use hospital ones as it would save her having to wash them and, also, it caused a lot of problems if patients' own pyjamas were mixed up in the hospital laundry'.

The nurse said this with such authority that the daughter did not like to argue that she would gladly do this for her father and it did not matter if they were lost. It mattered far more to her to see her father dressed in his own pyjamas, so that he looked like himself. She wanted to see him shaved and clean, his dentures in place and wearing his own clothes.

A few days after admission, John died. This left his daughter with the abiding memory of her father in a strange place wearing pyjamas that were not his.

This case study illustrates that, while there are quality measures based on agreed standards, patients and carers base their judgements on what they see as the essential elements of care. A study that explored patients' and nurses' perceptions of quality of nursing care, using a qualitative approach rather than a questionnaire, found that, while there were some differences in perception between patients and nurses, there was also some agreement (Redfern and Norman, 1999). Themes that were shared by both groups were to do with a therapeutic ward atmosphere and therapeutic, thorough and sensitive individualised care. *The nurse–patient relationship was central to the quality of nursing* (p416). This study also said it was important to take an interest in patients as individuals and treat them as partners. Many of the issues discussed earlier in the book are viewed by patients and carers as quality indicators.

Principles of nursing practice

To clarify the issue for nurses, patients and carers, the Royal College of Nursing has produced the *Principles of Nursing Practice* (RCN, 2010b), developed together with the Department of Health in England and patient groups. These principles define quality nursing care and also provide a framework to support the evaluation of care. Although it will be managers who apply this framework to practice, it does provide guidance for everyone about quality nursing care. You need to consider these principles alongside the NMC *Code* (2008a) and inspectorate standards. They are seen as overarching principles that describe for the public what they can expect from nursing in any setting, and apply to healthcare assistants, students and registered nurses. At a service level, evidence-based clinical guidelines are produced by the Guidelines and Audit Implementation Network (GAIN) in Northern Ireland, the Scottish Intercollegiate Guidelines Network (SIGN) and NICE in England and Wales. The RCN has produced a document describing eight principles, which you can read more about at **www.rcn.org.uk/development/practice/ principles**.

Principle D states that *Nurses and nursing staff provide and promote care that puts people at the centre, involves patients, service users, their families and their carers in decisions and helps them make informed choices about their treatment and care* (RCN, 2010a, p5). The way that you would decide whether this principle is applied would be to measure patient perception of their involvement in decision-making and their confidence in their nurses' skills and knowledge. You need, therefore, to reflect on your practice, as these RCN principles apply to you as a student. Reflect on your recent clinical experience and whether you feel you have followed this principle.

Essence of Care benchmarking

The *Essence of Care* benchmarks were first introduced in 2001 and were revised in 2010 (DH, 2010c). The aim of these benchmarks is to set a standard for high-quality care. They were developed through discussions with patients, carers and nurses, and are intended to determine best practice from the patient perspective, providing a structure for localised quality improvement. This means that they are designed to be used by practitioners in liaison with patients and carers to define and examine the quality of their own practice. The idea is that, if you are involved in defining what standards of care should be, you will have ownership of them and feel more motivated to achieve them. As this process of determining standards should involve patients and carers, it promotes patient-centred care and a shared vision of what care should be. The benchmarks have been designed to be universally applicable in healthcare. In other words, they are applicable to a wide range of care settings. As it is the practitioners in the care area defining the standard, they can make it relevant to their patient group.

Aspects of care

The aspects of care selected for benchmarking were those that had been identified as sources of concern. For example, one of the original aspects was food and drink. You may remember that there have been several reports expressing great concern about patients receiving their nutritional requirements, such as *Hungry to be Heard* (Age Concern, 2006). Pain management is the most recent addition to the topic areas and arose from public demand. The Department of Health (2010a) now lists benchmarks focused on 12 aspects of care:

* bladder, bowel and continence care;
* care environment;
* food and drink;
* prevention and management of pain;
* personal hygiene;
* prevention and management of pressure ulcers;
* promoting health and well-being;
* record keeping
* respect and dignity;
* safety;
* self-care.

Benchmarking

You may find this benchmarking framework for quality improvement in care easier to understand because it is based on a systematic process, with stages like those of the nursing process. Benchmarking is *A systematic process in which current practice and care are compared to, and amended to attain, best practice and care* (DH, 2010c, p9).

This means that the first stage is similar to what was discussed in relation to assessment. Thus, just as patient problems were identified, in benchmarking you need to establish which are priority areas of practice for improvement. This involves setting up a group of practitioners, nurses and patient representatives to think about which aspect of care, and any of the associated factors, are not being met or whether there are any complaints about this aspect of practice. This then needs to be appraised according to the patient-focused outcome and associated factors. If issues for improvement are identified, a plan for improvement needs to be drawn up and put in place. Following this, patients, carers and staff need to evaluate whether this aspect of care has improved and whether they are now happy that the outcome is being met. Once this has been achieved, practice can be reappraised to determine further areas where improvement is required.

Best practice should also be disseminated. *Energise for Excellence* (DH, 2010d) is a quality framework that aims to improve patient experience and quality. It is strategically positioned as the overarching approach to implementation of the *Essence of Care* and other government quality assurance initiatives. It also adopts a systematic approach in its cycle of continuous improvement and development.

Benchmarking practice

Each aspect of care has benchmark statements. These are overall patient-focused outcomes, which are statements of what patients and/or carers want from care, and they can be found in the *Essence of Care* toolkit (DH, 2010c). For each patient-focused outcome, there are factors that need to be appraised in order to evaluate whether the outcome has been achieved. In this appraisal, there are indicators to be considered. Some of these indicators have been defined in the document, while others should be determined by the people in the benchmarking group. To illustrate this, let's look at the aspect of self-care (remember we discussed this concept in Chapter 7). For self-care, the agreed patient-focused outcome is *People have control over their care* (DH, 2010a, p8), and the following factors for achievement need to be appraised:

- choice;
- assessment, planning, implementation, evaluation and revision of care;
- risk;
- knowledge and skills;
- partnership;
- access to services and resources;
- environment.

For each of these factors, a continuum of practice from poor to best is identified, and there are indicators for where practice sits on this continuum. The first factor for self-care is *choice*, and the continuum for poor to best practice for *choice* (DH, 2010a, p9) is shown below.

Poor practice ———————————————————————— **Best practice**

(People are not
given a choice on
how their care is
delivered)

(People are enabled
to make informed
choices about caring
for themselves and
those choices are
respected)

In deciding where their practice sits on this continuum, benchmarking groups use the indicators identified and any others they define. Examples of indicators from the *Essence of Care* for *choice* are *consistent information is provided by staff* and *evaluation and revision of care continues to reflect people's choices* (DH, 2010a, p9).

To understand this system more fully, it would be useful to try the following activity.

Activity 9.4 — *Decision-making*

If you can, find three friends to help you and then work in pairs for points 1 and 2. One pair should look at these from a nurse's viewpoint and the other pair should take a patient or carer perspective. The activity is based on factor 5 for self-care, which is *partnership* (DH, 2010a, p15).

1. Try to identify what you think is poor and what is best practice for *partnership*.
2. Place your suggestions on the continuum.

Poor practice ———————————————————— Best practice

continued opposite . . .

continued . . .

3. What indicators would you use to decide what the quality of partnership practice was in your area?
4. Now, compare your ideas with the other pair. Are there any similarities or differences? Pretend you are a benchmarking group and see if you as nurses and patients/carers can agree what the indicators should be.
5. Having agreed on indicators, what types of evidence about these would you collect in practice?

Outline answers are given at the end of the chapter.

While there are some suggestions for types of evidence given at the end of the chapter, you may have had some debate about the focus of these and how they would be collected. A useful framework for quality assurance by Donabedian (1980), which has been used in nursing, comprises the three elements of structure, process and outcome. *Structure* is about the relatively stable elements of the care setting, such as the number of qualified staff. *Process* concerns issues during care delivery, such as respect of patient autonomy, and *outcome* is a measure of achievement, such as a change in health behaviour. Evaluating care as discussed earlier would mean that thinking about the interventions was about process and goal achievement about outcome. While Donabedian viewed structure as the least important, he declared that there was a *fundamental, functional relationship amongst the three* (1980, p81). In other words, the relationship between them was such that poor-quality structural issues would impact on process and outcome.

Quality and patient satisfaction

Quality is not synonymous with patient satisfaction but it is a significant element of it. Several authors (Wagner and Bear, 2008; Walsh and Walsh, 1999) agree that nursing care plays a prominent role in patient satisfaction. It is clients, both as individuals and together, who define what quality means: client satisfaction is an important component of care (Donabedian, 1980). Using his own framework, Donabedian acknowledged that patients were probably more able to comment on interpersonal aspects of care than technical ones.

You may recall from Chapter 2 that, for the last decade, it has been government policy to conduct annual National Surveys of Patient and User Experience. The results of these surveys are used to monitor the performance of NHS organisations and as an overall measure of patient experience by the Department of Health. An annual report is produced by the Picker Institute on behalf of the Care Quality Commission. So you can see that, unlike *Essence of Care* benchmarking, which is at a local level, these are institutional appraisals, the results of which are available nationally. They judge quality in terms of waiting times and so on. To find out more about the National Surveys, try Activity 9.5.

While you were on the above website, you may have chosen to explore how these surveys were conducted. You will have discovered something about the methods used to obtain information on patient and carer perspectives. It is important to consider this information as it will have an impact on how you will decide what credence to give to the findings. This, of course, also applies to research studies.

Activity 9.6 was designed to start you thinking about the importance of the tools used to gather information and the differences in the data that they yield. The Patients Association (2010) pointed out that people who passed away would not be able to respond to the survey, and also that frail, elderly people are probably unable to respond. Therefore, the findings of in-patient surveys would not be representative of the patient population. Maybe these surveys should include carer feedback.

Measurement of patient satisfaction

When you conduct a survey on patient satisfaction, the results need to be measured in some way. Many of these surveys use Likert scales in which the respondent is asked to rank items on a scale from 'strongly agree' to 'strongly disagree'. Such instruments should have been tested for reliability and validity, but Campen et al. (1995), in their review of 113 such instruments, found that only 41 offered evidence of this testing. The Service Quality (SERVQUAL) instrument was found to have good internal consistency and did discriminate different dimensions of quality from the patient perspective. However, further work is necessary to develop an instrument that truly reflects the patient's perspective.

Patient satisfaction can be a measure of the process, or the outcome of care (Coulter and Ellins,2006); it is hard to use patient views to map trends because of the differences in patient experience and knowledge of healthcare, or their dependency on providers. There is an old adage that says *satisfaction [is] what the patient says it is*; if this is so, there will be many variations of it.

Because there are quite a few problems in collecting data by survey, there has been a shift towards collecting information about patient experiences through focus groups. These tend to elicit information about events that happened rather than rate care using evaluation categories. Questionnaires could be developed from issues raised by focus group participants. It is useful for managers to be able to pinpoint specific issues, such as if a high percentage of patients said it took more than 15 minutes for their call bell to be answered. Although it is good to hear when patients are pleased with their care, healthcare providers need to focus on the views of people who have negative experiences with healthcare so as to identify areas for improvement (Coyle and Williams, 2001). Chief among the negative reports are issues of power, control and the approachability of staff.

Complaints and advocacy

It may seem strange to think about complaints when talking about quality, but, as Coulter and Ellins (2006) suggested, if these were looked at collectively, they would offer insights as to how practice could be improved. Coyle and Williams (2001) found that people gave positive evaluations, even when they were unhappy with some elements of care. Why do you think this is? Activity 9.7 will encourage you to think about patient complaints.

Activity 9.7   *Reflection*

- Give reasons why a patient would not complain, even though they were unhappy with care.
- If a patient complains, how does this make you feel?

An outline answer is given at the end of the chapter.

Reflecting on how you feel about complaints is important because your feelings can influence your behaviour. Negative feelings may mean that you avoid dealing with the situation. You should also remember that patient and carer anxiety may manifest itself as dissatisfaction. If you take a little time to talk to people, you may be able to explore these anxieties and avoid a complaint. Just sitting by a patient's bed for five minutes to discuss their care improves patient satisfaction (Dingman et al., 1999, cited in Coyle and Williams, 2001). It helps patients feel empowered. Don't dismiss complaints such as a patient's hair being untidy or nails not being clean as being trivial and justify them by saying that you are too busy. Try to see this from the anxious relative's perspective and talk to them about their concerns and how these may be resolved.

- What should you do when a patient makes a complaint?
- Find out about your local policy on complaints and also how patients and carers can access information about the Patient Advisory and Liaison Service (PALS) in your clinical area.

An outline answer is given at the end of the chapter.

Ignoring complaints is not an option you should pursue. If all staff were to collate information about complaints, that would enable managers to identify areas of practice for improvement. If their complaints are ignored, patients tend to be less adherent to treatment and more likely to miss appointments. This, together with any litigation, increases costs to the NHS (Coyle and Williams, 2001). The second point in Activity 9.8 asked you to find out about PALS, which you may remember was mentioned in the section on *The NHS Plan* in Chapter 2 (page 28).

Patient Advisory and Liaison Service

PALS was established to improve patient services. Its main functions are:

- to provide help and speedy resolutions to problems;
- to facilitate access to independent advice and advocacy services;
- to supply information about the NHS and deal with other help-related enquiries;
- to act as a mechanism for feedback to the Trust, which can then help to promote change and improvement.

You can see, therefore, that PALS is an important organisation. It exists to help people to express their concerns and explore solutions without recourse to the formal complaints procedure. You need to be aware of PALS and inform patients and carers about it. However, PALS staff are employed by NHS Trusts, which means that people may want to seek more independent advice. In such cases, people should be referred to the Independent Complaints Advocacy Service (ICAS), which was set up in 2003 to help people decide whether to go ahead with a formal complaint.

Complaints procedure for England

Since 2009, the NHS established a simple procedure. There should be information available about the local complaints procedure in the Trusts and there may be a complaints manager. NHS Trusts should seek to resolve complaints locally in the first instance. If you are still not satisfied, you can take your complaint to the Health Service Ombudsman. This ombudsman is independent of the NHS and government. Studying the ombudsman's report provides further scope for Trusts regarding quality improvement. The Patients Association (2010), however, citing a report by the Alzheimer's Society, found that only 7 per cent of people who complained were satisfied with the outcome. The Patients Association, therefore, called for the immediate employment of *patient safeguarding champions* (2010, p4).

Government policy and quality

A First Class Service: Quality in the new NHS (DH, 1998) sought to make quality an integral part of the service. This white paper identified that quality would be achieved by working with patients and users in *partnership for quality*. In Chapter 2, we looked at the National Service Frameworks that this paper sought to introduce, and you may also recall that it also brought about NICE, the Commission for Health Improvement and NHS Patient Surveys. A further aspect not discussed then was clinical governance.

Clinical governance

The RCN defined clinical governance as an *umbrella term for everything that helps to maintain and improve standards* (2003, p7). It was designed to create a framework or structure that would help clinicians to coordinate all activity concerning quality enhancement. Involving patients and the public is an essential element of this. Clinical governance is about promoting partnership by empowering people to have a greater say in service provision. It was about changing culture and empowering staff to improve quality locally. Clinical governance encompasses activities such as clinical audit, but it also involves supporting staff in their development, promoting team working and evidence-based practice.

Care Quality Commission

In Activity 9.5, you accessed the CQC website and you may have read more about its work. The CQC replaced the Commission for Health Improvement and is the independent regulator of health and adult social care services in England. It also protects the interests of people whose rights are restricted under the Mental Health Act. The remit is to improve services, remedy bad practice and champion patients' rights. It inspects health and social care establishments to ensure that they meet the essential care standards and registers establishments, as well as monitoring and publishing reports on patient experience.

In *High Quality Care for All*, Lord Darzi reiterated that the place of quality was *at the heart of the NHS* (2008, p5). This report saw quality as involving not only clinical safety but also individualised care, and stated that high-quality care involved patients *being treated with compassion, dignity and respect* (ibid.). It made further recommendations for quality improvement, including expansion of the work of NICE to ascertain quality standards. NICE's clinical standard-setting priorities would be determined by a new National Quality Board. There was also to be a new Quality Observatory, which would focus on local quality improvements. Patients' own accounts of the quality of their experiences would be captured in new quality accounts, which all healthcare providers for the NHS were required to produce from April 2010.

Equity and Excellence (DH, 2010b) articulated the role of HealthWatch England in involving patients and carers. This was to be a consumer champion under the control of the CQC. A new NHS Outcomes Framework would be established and would centre on three quality domains:

- effectiveness of care;
- safety and treatment of patients;
- broader experience that patients have of the treatment and care they receive.

Indicators of these outcomes would be developed from the NICE quality standards, with each standard having specific indicators. A system for linking quality achievement to financial remuneration would be developed, including the creation of best-practice tariffs. There would be quality increments administered by the Commission for Quality and Innovation (CQUIN). This white paper intended to drive quality improvement by financial incentive. Patient feedback, obtained in quality accounts and part of local quality commissioning, would, therefore, have a financial impact on services.

Chapter summary

As you can see, quality is an elusive concept and not easy to measure, but it is the concern of all staff. Measuring care experience starts with the evaluation that you carry out with patients and carers. Capturing patient and carer experience means that you need to listen to what they are saying about their care. This then extends to clinical governance and to Trust and national measurement of quality, but, remember, *quality is at the heart of everything we do* (DH, 2010b, p2).

Activities: brief outline answers

Activity 9.1 Evaluating patient care (page 146)

- Evaluation can take place during handover, or at the patient's bedside.
- It could take place at end of shift, daily or all the time.
- Nurses, members of the multi-disciplinary team, patients and carers could all be involved.

Activity 9.3 Evaluating health information (page 148)

- You could pilot the leaflet with patients and/or carers prior to usage. You could include a tear-off comment section, ask patient groups or ask individual patients.
- You should consider content, presentation and accessibility, for example.

Activity 9.4 Essence of Care benchmarks (pages 152–3)

1. **Poor practice** ———————————————————— **Best practice**
   (People, carers, staff   (People, carers, staff
   and organisations do   and organisations
   not work in partnership)   work in partnership
                          to meet care needs)

   (DH, 2010a, p15)

2. Were these different between the pairs and could you agree?
3. Some indicators given in *Essence of Care* are about communication, documentation (shared contracts), partnership meetings, and how partnership arrangements are monitored and evaluated. Another

indicator is whether patients and carers are involved in staff education (DH, 2010a). You may have thought of some different local indicators.

5. Evidence could include patient and carer surveys, informal discussion, focus groups, letters of complaint or absence of these.

Activity 9.6 Feedback (page 154)

- **Questionnaire** – Advantages: can reach a large sample, wide geographical distribution, easy to analyse. Disadvantages: low response rates, respondents must be literate (remember Chapter 8), they lack depth, questions may be omitted. Also, it could be a different person responding or a group response.
- **Focus group** – Advantages: allows issues to be explored in depth, leader can clarify issues. Disadvantages: time-consuming, more difficult to analyse, needs to be well managed so that one group member does not dominate and all members' views are heard.
- **Other methods** – bedside terminals, kiosks, web-based surveys, hand-held devices, comment cards, mystery shoppers, PALS.

Activity 9.7 Patient complaints (page 155)

- They do not know how to complain, may not like to make a fuss, believe staff are doing their best, are afraid of reprisals, know they will have to use the service again, or think they should be grateful because the service is free.
- It may make you feel upset, defensive or inadequate.

Activity 9.8 Dealing with a complaint (page 156)

- As a student, you would take advice from your mentor, but you need to learn what should be done.
- Acknowledge that they are upset and ask if they have any specific concerns they want to talk about.
- Arrange to discuss these in a private place. Arrange a set time. See if they want someone senior to be present.
- Explore any concerns and discuss ways to remedy the situation. For example, if they feel that they have insufficient information, arrange for them to access this.
- If they are still unhappy, ask if they would like to use the advocacy service.
- Explain the complaints procedure.
- Record all your actions.

Further reading

Department of Health (DH) (2009) *Understanding What Matters: A guide to using patient feedback to transform services.* London: Department of Health.

This details how patient feedback can be accessed and utilised in quality improvement and indicates useful resources.

Department of Health (DH) (2010) *The Nursing Roadmap for Quality: A signposting map for nursing.* London: Department of Health.

This is a guide for quality and improvement, available online at **www.dh.gov.uk/cno**. It will help you to understand quality frameworks in relation to nursing practice and provides information about tools and resources.

Goodrich, J and Cornwell, J (2008) *Seeing the Person in the Patient: The Point of Care review paper.* London: King's Fund.

This examines care delivery from the patient and carer perspective and how care can be improved.

Royal College of Nursing (RCN) (2003) *Clinical Governance: An RCN resource guide.* London: RCN.

This is a comprehensive document on clinical governance and its usage in practice, including policy in all the home countries.

Useful websites

www.drfosterintelligence.co.uk

This is a public–private organisation that reports on quality and efficiency within the NHS. There is information about patient experience and engagement.

www.ic.nhs.uk

The Information Centre for Health and Social Care provides data on quality issues, including patient-reported outcome measures (PROMs).

www.institute.nhs.uk

The NHS Institute for Innovation and Improvement has a section on quality and value. There is also information about quality tools, including those for patient pathways.

www.nhssurveys.org

You can find reports on the NHS surveys here.

www.nice.org.uk

The National Institute for Health and Clinical Excellence which will detail its latest recommendations and guidelines.

www.pals.nhs.uk

This website provides much useful information for patient and carer advice and engagement, and includes a library. It also has details on the National PALS Network.

www.pickereurope.org

The Picker Institute Europe is an organisation whose function is to promote understanding of the patient's perspective in healthcare policy and practice. Much of its work is about research and evaluating patient experience. It undertakes NHS Patient Surveys for the CQC.

References

Age Concern (2006) *Hungry to be Heard*. London: Age Concern.

Ahnert, L, Pinquart, M and Lamb, ME (2006) Security of children's relationships with nonparental care providers: a meta-analysis. *Child Development*, 77(13): 664–79.

Allen, D (2000) Negotiating the role of expert carers on an adult hospital ward. *Sociology of Health and Illness*, 22(2): 149–71.

Arksey, H (2003) Scoping the field: services for carers with mental health problems. *Health and Social Care in the Community*, 11(4): 335–44.

Barber, P (1991) Caring: the nature of a therapeutic relationship, in Perry, A and Jolley, M (eds) *Nursing: A knowledge base for practice*. London: Edward Arnold.

Beasley, C (2010) Introduction, in Department of Health (DH), *The Nursing Roadmap for Quality: A signposting map for nursing*. Available online at at www.dh.gov.uk (accessed 2 December 2010).

Beresford, P (2005) 'Service user': regressive or liberatory terminology? *Disability & Society*, 20(4): 469–77.

Biley, F (1992) Some determinants that affect patient participation in decision-making about nursing care. *Journal of Advanced Nursing*, 17: 414–21.

Bowlby, J (1969, 1973, 1980) *Attachment and Loss*, vols I, II, III. London: Hogarth Press.

Bradburn, J (2003) Developments in user organisations, in Monroe, B and Oliviere, D (eds) *Patient Participation in Palliative Care*. Oxford: Oxford University Press.

Cahill, J (1998a) Patient participation – a review of the literature. *Journal of Advanced Nursing*, 7: 119–28.

Cahill, J (1998b) Patient's perceptions of bedside handovers. *Journal of Clinical Nursing*, 7: 351–9.

Campen, van C, Sixma, H, Friele, R, Kerseens, J and Peters, L (1995) Quality of care and patient satisfaction: a review of measuring instruments. *Medical Care Research & Review*, 52(1): 109–33.

Carers UK (2007a) *Real Change Not Short Change*. London: Carers UK.

Carers UK (2007b) *Valuing Carers: Calculating the value of unpaid care*. London: Carers UK.

Carers UK (2009) *Facts about Carers: Policy briefing*. Available online at www.carersuk.org (accessed 5 March 2010).

Carers UK (2010) *Equal Partners Briefing: Carers and the NHS*. Available online at www.carersuk/equalpartners (accessed 9 July 2010).

Caress, AL (2003) Giving information to patients. *Nursing Standard*, 17(43): 47–54.

Carper, BA (1978) Fundamental patterns of knowing in nursing. *Advances in Nursing Science*, 1: 13–23.

Cayton, H (2005) Quotation, in Department of Health (DH) *Supporting People with Long Term Conditions: An NHS and social care model to support local innovation and integration*. Available online at www.dh.gov.uk (accessed 2 October 2010).

Cayton, H (2008) Patients as entrepreneurs, in Dixon, A (ed.) *Engaging Patients in Their Health: How the NHS needs to change*. Report from the Sir Roger Bannister Health Summit, Leeds Castle, 17–18 May 2007. London: The King's Fund.

Chambers, D and Thompson, S (2008) Empowerment and its application in health promotion in acute care settings: nurses' perceptions. *Journal of Advanced Nursing*, 65(1): 130–8.

Clarke, A, Hanson, J and Ross, H (2003) Seeing the person behind the patient: enhancing the care of older people using a biographical approach. *Journal of Clinical Nursing*, 12: 697–706.

Clothier, C, MacDonald, A and Shaw, D (2004) *Independent Inquiry Relating to Deaths and Injuries on the Children's Ward at Grantham and Kesteven General Hospital* (the Clothier Report). London: The Stationery Office.

Concise Oxford English Dictionary (2010). Available online at www.askoxford.com/concise (accessed 27 June 2010).

Cook, T (2007) *The History of the Carers' Movement*. London: Carers UK.

Coulter, A (2002) *The Autonomous Patient: Ending paternalism in medical care*. London: The Stationery Office.

Coulter, A (2008) Patients as decision-makers, in Dixon, A (ed.) *Engaging Patients in Their Health: How the NHS needs to change*. Report from the Sir Roger Bannister Health Summit, Leeds Castle, 17–18 May 2007. London: The King's Fund.

Coulter, A and Ellins, J (2006) *Patient-focused Interventions: A review of the evidence*. London: Health Foundation.

Coulter, A, Entwistle, V and Gilbert, J (1998) *Informing Patients: An assessment of the quality of patient information materials*. London: The King's Fund.

Coyle, J and Williams, B (2001) Valuing people as individuals: development of an instrument through a survey of person-centredness in secondary care. *Journal of Advanced Nursing*, 36(3): 450–9.

Darzi, A (2007) *Our NHS, Our Future* (Interim Report). Available online at www.dh.gov.uk (accessed 20 October 2010).

Darzi, A (2008) *High Quality Care for All: NHS next stage review final report*. London: Department of Health. Available online at www.ournhs.nhs.uk (accessed 17 October 2010).

Davies, NJ (2010) Improving self-management for patients with long-term conditions. *Nursing Standard* 24(25): 49–56.

Deacon, M, Fitzpatrick, M and Presho, M (2008) Informal carers: valuing our assets, in Presho, M (ed.) *Managing Long Term Conditions: A social model for community practice*. Chichester: Wiley-Blackwell.

Deber, R, Kraetschmer, N, Urowitz, S and Sharpe, N (2005) Patient, consumer, client, or customer: what do people want to be called? *Health Expectations*, 8(4): 345–51.

Department for Children, Schools and Families (DCSF) (2003) *Every Child Matters*. London: DCSF.

Department of Health (DH) (1997) *The New NHS: Modern, dependable*. London: HMSO.

Department of Health (DH) (1998) *A First Class Service: Quality in the new NHS*. Available online at www.dh.gov.uk (accessed 26 November 2010).

Department of Health (DH) (1999a) *Caring for Carers*. Available online at www.dh.gov.uk (accessed 29 July 2010).

Department of Health (DH) (1999b) *Saving Lives: Our healthier nation*. London: HMSO.

Department of Health (DH) (1999c) *National Strategy for Carers: Caring for carers*. Available online at www.dh.gov.uk (accessed 29 July 2010).

Department of Health (DH) (1999d) *Better Care, Higher Standards: A charter for long term care*. Available online at www.dh.gov.uk (accessed 9 December 2010).

Department of Health (DH) (2000) *The NHS Plan: A plan for investment, a plan for reform*. London: HMSO.

Department of Health (DH) (2001a) *The Expert Patient: A new approach to chronic disease management for the 21st century*. Available online at www.dh.gov.uk/selfcare (accessed 10 October 2010).

Department of Health (DH) (2001b) *Shifting the Balance of Power: Securing delivery.* Available online at www.dh.gov.uk (accessed 9 December 2010).

Department of Health (DH) (2001c) *The Essence of Care: Patient-focused benchmarking for health care practitioners (revised 2003).* London. HMSO. Available online at www.dh.gov.uk/en/Publicationsandstatistics/ PublicationsPolicy And Guidance/DH_4005475 (accessed 21 March 2010).

Department of Health (DH) (2002) *Securing Our Future: Taking the long-term view* (The Wanless Report). Available online at www.dh.gov.uk (accessed 9 December 2010).

Department of Health (DH) (2003a) *Confidentiality: NHS code of practice.* London: HMSO.

Department of Health (DH) (2003b) *Toolkit for Producing Patient Information, Version 2.0.* Available online at www.dh.gov.uk (accessed 2 October 2010).

Department of Health (DH) (2004a) *Better Information, Better Choices, Better Health.* Available online at www.dh.gov.uk (accessed 2 March 2009).

Department of Health (DH) (2004b) *Building on the Best.* London: HMSO.

Department of Health (DH) (2004c) *Getting over the Wall: How the NHS is improving the patient's experience.* Available online at www.dh.gov.uk (accessed 9 December 2010).

Department of Health (DH) (2004d) *Securing Health for the Whole Population.* Available at www.dh.gov.uk (accessed 9 December 2010).

Department of Health (DH) (2004e) *The NHS Improvement Plan: Putting people at the heart of public services.* London: HMSO.

Department of Health (DH) (2005a) *Self Care: A real choice.* Available online at www.dh.gov.uk/ prod_consum_dh/groups/dh_digitalassets/@dh@en?documents?digitalasset/dh_4101702.pdf (accessed 8 October 2010).

Department of Health (DH) (2005b) *Public Attitudes to Self Care Baseline Survey: Executive summary.* Available online at www.dh.gov.uk (accessed 11 October 2010).

Department of Health (DH) (2005c) *Supporting People with Long-term Conditions: An NHS and social care model to support local innovation and integration.* Available online at www.dh.gov.uk (accessed 10 October 2010).

Department of Health (DH) (2005d) *Supporting Self Care – A Practical Option: Diagnostic, monitoring and assistive tools, devices, technologies and equipment to support self care: Summary of a review report.* Available online at www.dh.gov.uk (accessed 7 October 2010).

Department of Health (DH) (2005e) *Now I Feel Tall: What a patient-led NHS feels like.* Available online at www.dh.gov.uk (accessed 9 December 2010).

Department of Health (DH) (2006a) *Our Health, Our Care, Our Say: A new direction for community services.* Available online at www.dh.gov.uk (accessed 10 November 2010).

Department of Health (DH) (2006b) *A Stronger Local Voice: A framework for creating a stronger local voice in the development of health and social services.* Available at www.dh.gov.uk (accessed 9 December 2010).

Department of Health (DH) (2008a) *Your Health, Your Way: A guide to long-term conditions and self care.* Available online at www.dh.gov.uk/yourhealth (accessed 10 February 2011).

Department of Health (DH) (2008b) *Carers at the Heart of 21st-century Families and Communities: 'A caring system on your side. A life of your own'.* London: HMSO.

Department of Health (DH) (2008c) *NHS Choices: Delivering for the NHS.* Available online at www.dh.gov.uk (accessed 7 December 2010).

Department of Health (DH) (2009a) *Putting Patients at the Heart of Care: the vision for patient and public engagement in health and social care*. Available online at www.dh.gov.uk (accessed 7 December 2010).

Department of Health (DH) (2009b) *The NHS Constitution*. Available online at www.dh.gov.uk (accessed 20 December 2010).

Department of Health (DH) (2010a) *Essence of Care 2010: Benchmarks for self care*. Available online at www.dh.gov.uk (accessed 26 November 2010).

Department of Health (DH) (2010b) *Equity and Excellence: Liberating the NHS*. Available online at www.dh.gov.uk (accessed 8 October 2010).

Department of Health (DH) (2010c) *Essence of Care 2010: Benchmarks for promoting health*. London: The Stationery Office. Available online at www.dh.gov.uk (accessed 26 November 2010).

Department of Health (DH) (2010d) *Energise for Excellence (E4E)*. Available online at www.dh.gov.uk/cno (accessed 2 December 2010).

Dewar, A and Morse, J (1995) Unbearable incidents: failure to endure the experience of illness. *Journal of Advanced Nursing*, 22: 957–64.

Dingwall, R, Rafferty, AM and Webster, C (1991) *An Introduction to the Social History of Nursing*. London: Routledge.

Dixon, A and Dickson, N (2008) Next steps in patient and public engagement, in Dixon, A (ed.) *Engaging Patients in Their Health: How the NHS needs to change*. London: The King's Fund.

Donabedian, A (1980) *Explorations in Quality Assessment and Monitoring, vol. 1: The definition of quality and approaches to its assessment*. Ann Arbor, MI: Administration Press.

Dougherty, L and Lister, S (2008) *The Royal Marsden Hospital Manual of Clinical Nursing Procedures* (7th edition). Oxford: Blackwell Publishing.

Edwards, M, Hill, S and Edwards, A (2009) Health literacy – achieving consumer 'empowerment' in health care decisions, in Edwards, A and Elwyn, G (eds) *Shared Decision-making in Health Care: Achieving evidence-based patient choice*. Oxford: Oxford University Press.

Elliot-Cannon, C (1990) Mental handicap and nursing models, in Salvage, J and Kershaw, B (eds) *Models for Nursing 2*. London: Scutari.

Entwistle, V, Watt, I and Sowden, A (1997) Information to facilitate patient involvement in decision-making – some issues. *Journal of Clinical Effectiveness*, 2(3): 69–72.

Farrell, C, Towle, A and Godolphin, W (eds) (2006) *Where's the Patient's Voice in Health Professional Education?* A report from the 1st international conference organised by the Division of Health Care Communication, University of British Columbia.

Ford, P and Walsh, M (1994) *New Rituals for Old: Nursing through the looking glass*. London: Butterworth-Heinemann.

Frank, J and Mclarnon, J (2008) *Principles of Practice for Young Carers and their Families*. London: The Children's Society. Available online at www.youngcarer.com/showPage.php?file=index.htm (accessed 10 August 2010).

Gallagher, A and Seedhouse, D (2002) Dignity in Care: the views of patients and relatives. *Nursing Times*, 98(43): 39–40.

Gallant, M, Beaulieu, M and Carnevale, F (2002) Partnership: an analysis of the concept within the nurse–client relationship. *Journal of Advanced Nursing*, 40: 149–57.

Garratt, E (2009) *The Key Findings Report for the 2008 Inpatient Survey*. Oxford: Acute Co-ordination Centre for the NHS Patient Survey Programme, Picker Institute Europe. Available online at www.nhssrveys.org/Filestore//documents/Key_findings_report_for_the_2008_Inpatient_Survey.pdf (accessed 2 March 2011).

Gibson, C (1991) A concept analysis of empowerment. *Journal of Advanced Nursing*, 16: 354–61.

Gilbert, J (2006) Overview, in Farrell, C, Towle, A and Godolphin, W (eds) *Where's the Patient's Voice in Health Professional Education?* A report from the 1st international conference organised by the Division of Health Care Communication, University of British Columbia.

Glaser, B and Strauss, AL (1967) *The Discovery of Grounded Theory: Strategies for qualitative research*. Chicago, IL: Aldine.

Glasper, EA and Richardson, J (eds) (2006) *A Textbook of Children's and Young People's Nursing*. London: Elsevier.

Goffman, I (1961) *Asylums: Essays on social situations of mental patients and other inmates*. Garden City, NY: Doubleday.

Goodrich, J and Cornwell, J (2008) *Seeing the Person in the Patient: The Point of Care review paper*. London: The King's Fund. Available online at www.kingsfund.org.uk/publications (accessed 10 January, 2011).

Gray, N (2009) Health literacy is not just reading and writing. *The Pharmaceutical Journal*, 283: 333–6.

Gray, R and Robson, D (2002) Medication management for people with a diagnosis of schizophrenia. *Nursing Times*, 98(47): 38–41. Available online at www.nursingtimes.net/nursing-practice-clinical-reserach/medication-managment (accessed 25 October 2010).

Grime, J, Blenkinsopp, A, Raynor, D, Pollock, K and Knapp, P (2007) The role and value of written information for patients about individual medicines: a systematic review. *Health Expectations*, 10(3): 286–98.

Haddock, J (1996) Towards further clarification of the concept of 'dignity'. *Journal of Advanced Nursing*, 24(95): 924–31.

Hall, ET (1966) *The Hidden Dimension: Man's use of space in public and private*. Garden City, NY: Doubleday.

Hart, M (1996) Incorporating outpatient perceptions into definitions of quality. *Journal of Advanced Nursing*, 24: 1234–40.

Hasman, A, Coulter, A and Askham, J (2006) *Education for Partnership: Developments in medical education*. Oxford: Picker Institute Europe.

Hemphill, AI and Dearmum, AK (2006) Working with children and families, in Glasper, EA and Richardson, J (eds) *A Textbook of Children's and Young People's Nursing*. London: Elsevier.

Henderson, S (2003) Power imbalance between nurses and patients: a potential inhibitor of partnership in care. *Journal of Clinical Nursing*, 12: 501–8.

Hewison, A (1995) Nurses' power in interactions with patients. *Journal of Advanced Nursing*, 21: 75–82.

Hewitt-Taylor, J (2005) Caring for children with complex and continuing health needs. *Nursing Standard*, 19(42): 41–7.

Hickey, G and Kipping, C (1998) Exploring the concept of user involvement in mental health through a participation continuum. *Journal of Clinical Nursing*, 7: 83–8.

Hinchliff, S, Norman, S and Schober, J (1998) *Nursing Practice and Health Care*. London: Arnold.

Hirst, M (2005) Carer distress: a prospective, population-based study. *Social Science & Medicine*, 61: 697–708.

HM Government (2010) *Working Together to Safeguard Children: A guide to inter-agency working to safeguard and promote the welfare of children*. Available online at http://publications.education.gov.uk/eOrderingDownload/00305-2010DOM-EN-v3.pdf (accessed 2 March 2011).

Hogston, R and Marjoram, P (2007) *Foundations of Nursing Practice: Leading the way*. London: Palgrave Macmillan.

Hogston, R and Simpson, P (2007) *Foundations of Nursing Practice: Making the difference*. London: Palgrave Macmillan.

Holt, J, Coates, C, Cotterill, D, Eastburn, S, Laxton, J, Mistry, H and Young, C (2010) Identifying common competence in health and social care: an example of multi-institutional and inter-professional working. *Nurse Education Today*, 30: 264–70.

Hook, M (2006) Partnering with patients – a concept ready for action. *Journal of Advanced Nursing*, 56: 133–43.

House of Commons (2007) *The Health Committee's Report on Patient and Public Involvement in the NHS*. London: The Stationery Office.

Involve (2010) *Supporting Public Involvement in NHS, Public Health and Social Care Research*. London: National Institute for Health Research.

Jewell, S (1994) Patient participation: what does it mean to nurses? *Journal of Advanced Nursing*, 19: 433–8.

Johns, C (1991) The Burford Nursing Development Unit holistic model of nursing practice. *Journal of Advanced Nursing*, 16: 1090–8.

Jones, A and Collins, S (2007) Nursing assessments and other tasks: influences on participation in interaction between patients and nurses, in Collins, S, Britten, N, Ruusuvuori, J and Thompson, A (2007) *Patient Participation in Health Care Consultations*. Milton Keynes: Open University Press.

Jones, M, O'Neill, P, Waterman, H and Webb, C (1997) Building a relationship: communications and relationships between staff and stroke patients on a rehabilitation ward. *Journal of Advanced Nursing*, 26: 101–10.

Keen, A and Lewis, I (2008) Foreword, in *Common Core Principles to Support Self Care*. Leeds: Skills for Care and Skills for Health.

Kerr, M (2002) A qualitative study of shift handover practice and function from a socio-technical perspective. *Journal of Advanced Nursing*, 37: 125–34.

Kralik, D, Koch, T and Wotton, K (1997) Engagement and detachment: understanding patients' experiences in nursing. *Journal of Advanced Nursing*, 26: 399–407.

Lackey, N and Gates, M (2001) Adults' recollections of their experiences as young caregivers of family members with chronic physical illnesses. *Journal of Advanced Nursing*, 34(3): 320–8.

Latimer, J (2000) *The Conduct of Care*. London: Blackwell Science.

Llewellyn, A and Hayes, S (2008) *Fundamentals of Nursing Care: A textbook for students of nursing and healthcare*. Glasgow: Reflect Press.

Luker, K, Austin, L, Caress, A and Hallett, C (2000) The importance of 'knowing the patient': community nurses' constructions of quality in providing palliative care. *Journal of Advanced Nursing*, 31(4): 775–82.

Manley, K, Hardy, S, Titchen, A, Garbett, R and McCormack, B (2005) *Changing Patients' Worlds through Nursing Practice Expertise: A Royal College of Nursing research report, 1998–2004*. London: RCN. Available online at www.rcn.org.uk/_data/assets/pdf_file/0005/78647/002512.pdf (accessed 2 March 2011).

Marks-Maran, D (1992) Rethinking the nursing process, in Jolley, M and Brykczynska, G (eds) *Nursing Care: The challenge to change*. London: Edward Arnold.

Marland, G and Marland, C (2000) Power dressing. *Nursing Times*, 96(9): 30–1.

Marteau, T (2009) Informed choice: a construct in search of a name, in Edwards, A and Elwyn, G (2009) *Shared Decision-making in Health Care: Achieving evidence-based patient choice*. Oxford: Oxford University Press.

Martens, K (1998) An ethnographic study of the process of medication discharge education (MDE). *Journal of Advanced Nursing*, 27: 341–8.

Mason, T and Whitehead, E (2003) *Thinking Nursing*. Milton Keynes: Open University Press.

McCaughan, E and Thompson, K (2000) Information needs of cancer patients receiving chemotherapy at a day-case unit in Northern Ireland. *Journal of Clinical Nursing*, 9: 851–8.

McCormack, B and McCance, T (2006) Development of a framework for person-centred nursing. *Journal of Advanced Nursing*, 56: 472–9.

McGarry, J and Arthur, A (2001) Informal caring in late life: a qualitative study of older carers. *Journal of Advanced Nursing*, 33(2): 182–9.

McQueen, A (2000) Nurse–patient relationships and partnership in hospital care. *Journal of Clinical Nursing*, 9: 723–31.

McQueen, A (2004) Emotional intelligence in nursing work. *Journal of Advanced Nursing*, 47: 101–8.

Menzies, IEP (1960) A case study in the functioning of social systems as a defence against anxiety. *Human Relations*, 13: 95–121.

Miller, R (2000) *Researching Life Stories and Family Histories*. London: Sage.

Morrison, P (1994) *Understanding Patients*. London: Bailliere Tindall.

Morse, J (1991) Negotiating commitment and involvement in the nurse–patient relationship. *Journal of Advanced Nursing*, 16: 455–68.

Muetzel, AP (1988) Therapeutic nursing, in Pearson, A (ed.) *Primary Nursing*. London: Chapman Hall.

Mumford, M (1997) A descriptive study of the readability of patient information leaflets designed by nurses. *Journal of Advanced Nursing*, 26: 985–91.

Murray, E (2009) The role of internet-delivered interventions in self-care, in Edwards, A and Elwyn, G (2009) *Shared Decision-making in Health Care: Achieving evidence-based patient choice*. Oxford: Oxford University Press.

Murray, M and Atkinson, D (2000) *Understanding the Nursing Process* (6th edition). New York: McGraw Hill.

Naidoo, J and Wills, J (2001) *An Introduction to Health Studies*. Basingstoke: Palgrave.

National Assembly for Wales (2001) *Improving Health in Wales: A plan for the NHS with its partners*. Cardiff: National Assembly for Wales.

National Health Service (NHS) (2008) *NHS Choices: Delivering for the NHS*. Available online at www.nhs.uk (accessed 27 October 2010).

National Primary Care Research & Development Centre (2006) *Executive Summary, National Evaluation of the Expert Patients Programmes*. Available online at www.expertpatients.nhs.uk (accessed 20 September 2010).

Nightingale, F (1859) *Notes on Nursing – What it is and what it is not*. London: Duckworth.

Nolan, M and Dellasega, C (2000) 'I really feel I've let him down': supporting family carers during long-term care placement for elders. *Journal of Advanced Nursing*, 31(4): 75–67.

Nursing and Midwifery Council (NMC) (2002) *Practitioner–Client Relationships and the Prevention of Abuse*. London: NMC.

Nursing and Midwifery Council (NMC) (2008a) *The Code: Standards of conduct, performance and ethics for nurses and midwives*. London: NMC.

Nursing and Midwifery Council (2008b) *Standards for Medicine Management*. London: NMC.

Nursing and Midwifery Council (NMC) (2010a) *Standards for Pre-registration Nursing Education*. London: NMC.

Nursing and Midwifery Council (NMC) (2010b) *Guidance on Professional Conduct for Nursing and Midwifery Students*. London: NMC.

Nutbeam, D (1998) *Health Promotion Glossary.* Geneva: WHO.

Nutbeam, D (2000) Health literacy as a public health goal: a challenge for contemporary health education and communication strategies into the 21st century. *Health Promotion International*, 15(3): 259–67.

Office of National Statistics (ONS) (2001) *Census 2001.* London: HMSO.

Orem, D (1985) *Nursing: Concepts of practice* (3rd edition). New York: McGraw Hill.

Orem, D (2001) *Nursing: Concepts of practice* (6th edition). London: Mosby.

Orlando, M (1961) *The Dynamic Nurse–Patient Relationship.* New York: Putman.

Ostman, M and Hansson, L (2004) Appraisal of caregiving, burden and psychological distress in relatives of psychiatric inpatients. *European Psychiatry*, 19: 402–7.

Patients Association (2010) *Listen to Patients, Speak Up for Change.* Available online at at www.patients-association.org.uk (accessed 2 December 2010).

Paterson, B (2002) Practitioners' actions inhibited patient participation in self care decision making. *Evidence Based Nursing*, 5: 62.

Pearson, A (1989) *Primary Nursing: Nursing in the Burford and Oxford Nursing Development Units.* London: Chapman Hall.

Pearson, A and Vaughn, B (1986) *Nursing Models for Practice.* Oxford: Heinemann Nursing.

Pearson, A, Vaughn, B and Fitzgerald, M (2005) *Nursing Models for Practice.* Oxford: Heinemann.

Peplau, H (1952) *Interpersonal Relations in Nursing.* New York: Putman's Sons.

Perakyla, A, Ruusuvuori, J and Lindors, P (2007) What is patient participation? Reflections arising from the study of general practice, homoeopathy and psychoanalysis, in Collins, S, Britten, N, Ruusuvuori, J and Thompson, A (eds) *Patient Participation in Health Care Consultations.* Milton Keynes: Open University Press.

Pickard, S, Jacobs, S and Kirk, S (2003) Challenging professional roles: lay carers' involvement in health care in the community. *Social Policy & Adminstration*, 37: 82–96.

Picker Institute (2007) *At a Crossroads Without Signposts: The struggle to access information about health and social services.* London: Picker Institute.

Radwin, L (1996) 'Knowing the patient': a review of research on an emerging concept. *Journal of Advanced Nursing*, 23: 1142–6.

Redfern, S and Norman, I (1999) Quality of nursing care perceived by patients and their nurses: an application of critical incident technique. Part 2. *Journal of Clinical Nursing*, 8(4): 414–21.

Rempel, GR, Neufeld, A and Kushner, KE (2007) Interactive use of genograms and ecomaps in family caregiving research. *Journal of Family Nursing*, 13: 403–19.

Richards, N and Coulter, A (2007) *Is the NHS Becoming More Patient-Centred? Trends from national surveys of NHS patients in England 2002–07.* Oxford: Picker Institute Europe. Available online at www.pickereurope.org (accessed 2 March 2011).

Robbins, MA, McCluskey, HJ and Dedmen, J (2009) Safeguarding the adults, in Glasper A, McEwing, G and Richardson, J (eds) *Foundation Studies for Caring.* Basingstoke: Palgrave Macmillan.

Robertson, J (1955) Young children in long term hospitals. *Nursing Times*, 23: 63–5.

Robertson, J and Robertson, J (1970) *Separation and the Very Young.* London. Free Association Books.

Robertson, J and Robertson, J (1967–71) *Young Children in Brief Separation* (a series of five films). Robertson Films.

Rogers, A (2009) Developing expert patients, in Edwards, A and Elwyn, G (2009) *Shared Decision-making in Healthcare: Achieving evidence-based patient choice*. Oxford: Oxford University Press.

Roper, N, Logan, W and Tierney, A (2000) *The Roper, Logan and Tierney Model of Nursing*. London: Churchill Livingstone.

Royal College of Nursing (RCN) (2003a) *Defining Nursing*. London: RCN. Available online at www.rcn.org.uk (accessed 21 March, 2010).

Royal College of Nursing (RCN) (2003b) *Clinical Governance: An RCN resource guide*. London: RCN.

Royal College of Nursing (RCN) (2008) *Dignity for All*. London: RCN.

Royal College of Nursing (RCN) (2010a) A matter of principle. *RCN Bulletin*, 263: 5.

Royal College of Nursing (RCN) (2010b) *Principles of Nursing Practice*. Available online at www.rcn.org/development/practice/principles (accessed 23 November 2010).

Scottish National Executive (2000) *Our National Health: A plan for action, a plan for change*. Edinburgh: Scottish Executive Health Department.

Scovell, S (2010) Role of nurse-to-nurse handover in patient care. *Nursing Standard*, 24: 35–9.

Sharma, V, Whitney, D, Kazarian, SS and Manchanda, R (2000) Preferred terms for users of mental health services among service providers and recipients. *Psychiatric Services*, 51(2): 203–9.

Shuttleworth, A (2004) Improving drug concordance in patients with chronic conditions. *Nursing Times*, 100(24): 28–9.

Skills for Care and Skills for Health (2008) *Common Core Principles to Support Self Care: A guide to support implementation*. Leeds: Skills for Care and Skills for Health.

Smith, E, Ross, F, Donovan, S, Manthorpe, J, Brearley, S, Sitzia, J and Beresford, P (2008) Service user involvement in nursing, midwifery and health visiting research: a review of evidence and practice. *International Journal of Nursing Studies*, 45: 298–315.

Smith, L, Coleman, V and Bradshaw, M (eds) (2002) *Family Centred Care: Concept, theory and practice*. Basingstoke: Palgrave.

Smith, R and Draper, P (1994) Who is in control? An investigation of nurse and patient beliefs relating to control of their health care. *Journal of Advanced Nursing*, 19: 884–92.

Stein-Parbury, J (2000) *Patient and Person: Developing interpersonal skills*. London: Harcourt.

Stein-Parbury, J (2009) *Patient and Person. Developing interpersonal skills* (4th edition). London: Harcourt.

Stratford, M (2003) Palliative nursing, in Monroe, B and Oliviere, D (eds) *Patient Participation in Palliative Care*. Oxford: Oxford University Press.

Street, C and Powell, C (2008) Empowering patients: the role of the Expert Patient Programme in promoting health amongst those with long term conditions, in Presho, M (ed.) *Managing Longterm Conditions: A social model for community practice*. Chichester: Wiley Blackwell.

Sully, P and Dallas, J (2005) *Essential Communication Skills for Nurses*. Edinburgh: Elsevier Mosby.

Swanson, K (1991) Empirical development of a middle range theory of caring. *Nursing Research*, 40(3): 161–6.

Thompson, A (2007) The meaning of patient involvement and participation in healthcare consultations, in Collins, S, Britten, N, Ruusuvuori, J and Thompson, A (eds) *Patient Participation in Health Care Consultations*. Milton Keynes: Open University Press.

Timonen, L and Sihvonen, M (2000) Patient participation in bedside reporting on surgical wards. *Journal of Clinical Nursing*, 9: 542–8.

Trnobranski, P (1994) Nurse–patient negotiation: assumption or reality? *Journal of Advanced Nursing*, 19: 733–7.

von Wagner, C, Knight, K, Steptoe, A and Wardle, J (2007) Functional health literacy and health promoting behaviour in a national sample of British adults. *Journal of Epidemiology and Community Health*, 61: 1086–90.

Wagner, D and Bear, M (2008) Patient satisfaction with nursing care: a concept analysis within a nursing framework. *Journal of Advanced Nursing*, 65(3): 692–701.

Walker, E and Dewar, B (2001) How do we facilitate carers' involvement in decision-making? *Journal of Advanced Nursing*, 34(3): 329–37.

Walsh, K and Kowanko, I (2002) Nurses' and patients' perceptions of dignity. *International Journal of Nursing Practice*, 8(3): 143–51.

Walsh, M (1998) *Models and Critical Pathways in Clinical Nursing: Conceptual frameworks for care planning.* London: Bailliere Tindall.

Walsh, M and Walsh, A (1999) Measuring patient satisfaction with nursing care: experience of using the Newcastle Satisfaction with Nursing Scale. *Journal of Advanced Nursing*, 29(2): 307–15.

Warne, T and McAndrew, S (2007) Passive patient or engaged espert? Using a Ptolemaic approach to enhance mental health nurse education and practice. *International Journal of Mental Health Nursing*, 16: 224–9.

Warwick, M, Gallagher, R, Chenoweth, L and Stein-Parbury, J (2010) Self-management and symptom monitoring among older adults with chronic obstructive airway disease. *Journal of Advanced Nursing*, 66(4): 784–93.

Waterworth, S and Luker, K (1990) Reluctant collaborators: do patients want to be involved in decisions concerning care? *Journal of Advanced Nursing*, 15: 971–6.

Whittington, D and McLaughlin, C (2000) Finding time for patients: an exploration of nurses' time allocation in an acute psychiatric setting. *Journal of Psychiatric and Mental Health Nursing*, 7: 259–68.

Wilkinson, C and McAndrew, S (2008) 'I'm not an outsider, I'm his mother!' A phenomenological enquiry into carer experiences of exclusion from acute psychiatric settings. *International Journal of Mental Health Nursing*, 17: 392–401.

Williams, A (2001a) A literature review on the concept of intimacy in nursing. *Journal of Advanced Nursing*, 33(5): 660–7.

Williams, A (2001b) A study of practising nurses' perceptions and experiences of intimacy within the nurse-patient relationship. *Journal of Advanced Nursing*, 35: 188–96.

Wilson, H (2001) Power and partnership: a critical analysis of the surveillance discourses of child health nurses. *Journal of Advanced Nursing*, 36: 294–301.

Wollin, J, Yates, P and Kristjanson, L (2006) Supportive and palliative care needs identified by multiple sclerosis patients and their families. *International Journal of Palliative Nursing*, 12: 20–6.

Index